Pure Politics and Impure Science

Arthur M. Silverstein *is Professor of Ophthalmic Immunology and Occupant of the Independent Order of Odd Fellows Research Chair in Ophthalmology at The Johns Hopkins University School of Medicine.*

PURE POLITICS
AND IMPURE SCIENCE
The Swine Flu Affair

Arthur M. Silverstein

THE JOHNS HOPKINS UNIVERSITY PRESS
Baltimore and London

For Fran, Alison, Mark, and Judy

This book has been brought to publication with the generous assistance of the Andrew W. Mellon Foundation

The Johns Hopkins University Press, Baltimore, Maryland 21218
The Johns Hopkins Press Ltd., London

Library of Congress Cataloging in Publication Data

Silverstein, Arthur M.
    Pure politics and impure science.

    Bibliography: pp. 171-72
    Includes index.
    1. Swine influenza — Preventive inoculation — Political aspects — United States. 2. Swine influenza — United States — Preventive inoculation. 3. Medical policy — United States. I. Title
RA644.I6S54   614.5'18   81-47590
ISBN 0-8018-2632-2   AACR2

Table of Contents

Preface

I T is one of the hallowed traditions of the academic life that a university professor expects, and in some institutions is encouraged, to take a sabbatical year. The purpose of this leave of absence is sometimes to go elsewhere to learn new approaches to one's chosen field of study, sometimes to branch out into a completely new field, sometimes to engage in a scholarly pursuit such as writing a book, and occasionally simply to "recharge one's intellectual batteries." During my previous sabbatical leave in 1960-61, the irrepressible ambitions of youth led me to spend my time at a medical school in England, learning new approaches to my chosen scientific discipline of immunity and allergic diseases. This experience not only changed the direction of my scientific research, but provided fourteen years of such exciting and satisfying experimental work that I had no desire to desert it for another sabbatical leave of absence.

But even the most stimulating research project can pall after so long a period of time, and by late 1974 I had begun to think more and more seriously that another sabbatical leave was in order. I was now, however, neither as young nor as ambitious as I had been the first time, so I decided that it did not make any sense to go off somewhere to try to make a fresh start in a new scientific discipline: any other field would already be over-populated with bright and well-trained young scientists against whom I would suffer a tremendous competitive disadvantage. Equally, it did not appear logical to go off to some other laboratory to continue my work in the same field, for nowhere else could I function as efficiently on these problems as in my own shop. And finally, I did not yet feel ready to retire from the fray, to don the robes of scientific elder statesman, and to write the "definitive tome" in my scientific specialty.

I was thus faced with two choices: either give up the thought of a sabbatical and go back to my now somewhat stale routine, or find something completely new and different to do for a sabbatical year. All through 1974 I pondered this problem without finding a solution, until one day I chanced to see a public affairs announcement in the journal of the Federation of American Societies for Experimental Biology (FASEB).

This brief announcement invited applications from qualified scientists for a new program that FASEB planned to initiate the following year, a program aimed at placing a biologist in Congress as a Congressional Science Fellow. For many years the scientific community had criticized Congress for its lack of scientific expertise in dealing with the increasingly more complicated laws required by this age of science and high technology. To help meet this need, the American Association for the Advancement of Science had initiated a fellowship program to place scientists and engineers at the disposal of members of Congress and congressional committees, so that they might not only assist the Congress in dealing with complicated scientific issues but also help the scientific community to understand the legislative process and how public policy is made. Now, with FASEB's new program, experimental biology would be formally represented for the first time. I had scarcely finished reading this announcement, when I knew that this was what I wanted to do. That night I discussed it with my wife, and the next day sent off for an application. By March of 1975, I knew that I would be spending a year working in Congress, starting the following September.

I felt fortunate in being accepted on the staff of the Senate Health Subcommittee, chaired by Senator Edward M. Kennedy of Massachusetts. Here, I felt, was where the action was in biomedical research legislation, and here, I was sure, was where I could best bring to bear my twenty-odd years of scientific background and my knowledge of scientific objectivity and of the scientific method. With the advantage of my profound scientific insights, I felt sure that Senator Kennedy and I would have little difficulty in solving *any* problems that might exist in the biomedical arena. Given the jurisdiction of the Senate Health Subcommittee over all authorizing legislation in the Health segment of the Department of Health, Education, and Welfare (HEW), the Kennedy Health Subcommittee appeared to provide an admirable vehicle for me to help rationalize and consolidate the extensive biomedical research activities at the National Institutes of Health (among other problems with which I hoped to become involved). It was no wonder that my sense of excitement and anticipation grew as the September starting date neared.

Never were innocent expectations so abruptly upset by reality than were mine during the first days and weeks of my work with the Senate Health Subcommittee. The culture shock that accompanied my first exposure to the workings of the Senate was almost beyond description. The least of my problems was learning a completely new set of mechanical and procedural problems, such as how to organize a subcommittee hearing for Senator Kennedy; how to get the assistance of the subcommittee counsel or the Senate's legislative counsel to draft an amendment or a bill;

how to consult the Senate parliamentarian on the form and wording necessary to call up an amendment; how to bring a bill for consideration before the subcommittee and full committee and then report it to the full Senate; how to arrange with the Majority Leader's staff to get a bill on the Senate's calendar; and a hundred other similar items. For such matters I could rely upon the guidance of Leroy Goldman, staff director of the Health subcommittee, and on the other staff members of the subcommittee. The Kennedy staff had a reputation throughout the Senate as a tough, cocky, but extremely competent group, and they collectively took me under their benevolent wing from the start, giving me an invaluable education in the legislative process.

It was other aspects, however, of the way in which Congress functioned that I found so shocking and foreign to anything I had experienced before. First, there was the almost incomprehensible, frenetic pace of activity in the Senate's business, and the short attention span that could be devoted to any individual item. When some scientific question had come up in my previous life, I could afford to give it all the time it required: to think about what to do, to plan and carry out experiments, to confirm and reconfirm results, and only when I was absolutely convinced, finally to prepare a scientific paper for publication — a sequence of events that might last from months to years. In the Senate, by contrast, an idea for a bill, or an amendment to a bill, might have to be translated into legislative language and acted upon within days, or even hours, because of the constraints imposed by the schedule of the Senator, the subcommittee, the full committee, or the Senate itself. Then there were the large number of both routine and emergency activities that required the attention of every staff member. Each staffer was expected to keep moving along from six to ten major and minor issues, involving consultation with outside experts and with other Senate staffers; hearings, markups, actions on the floor of the Senate, coordinations with other staffers on the House side and also with appropriate bureaus in the executive branch — all of which overlapped and came in no logical order. Interspersed in this would be the need to answer calls or to see personally a variety of lobbyists, to answer letters from Senator Kennedy's constituents in Massachusetts, to write a speech for the Senator or to brief him for a television interview, to help prepare a letter to the Secretary of HEW on some other issue, and so on. It seemed that no sooner was it possible to begin work on an important issue than another one, even more urgent, demanded the immediate attention of the congressional staffer, so that the dozens of different issues active within the subcommittee and the hundreds of different issues active at any time within the Senate made it difficult to do full justice to anything. Looking back, I find it difficult to understand how any juggler could have kept so many balls in the air simultaneously and over so long a period of time, and how anything was ever accomplished under these conditions.

The greatest shock of all, however, was the necessity of reaching a decision and acting before all the facts were known and had been carefully analyzed. When the bell rings in the Senate corridors announcing that a vote is being held on the floor of the Senate, as occurs several hundred times during a session, then (ready or not) the Senator must go down to the floor and cast his vote, whether it is on a question of biomedical research, a complicated tax bill, the authorization of a missile system for the military, the approval of a Cabinet appointee, or the thousands of other issues that confront a complex society such as ours. No member of Congress, not even with the best staff, can be expert in all of these areas. Even when a senator has specialized in a subject, as Kennedy has in health, many questions arise in which the issues are not clear and about which reasonable people may differ — not only about the solution to the problem but even about whether the problem exists at all. And yet, when the bell rings to vote, despite the uncertainties, and despite the other preoccupations of both the staff and its senator, firm recommendations must be made on a course of action. Furthermore, these recommendations cannot be couched in vague terms or in terms of "on the one hand" and "on the other hand," but in terms of yes or no — as though every important societal issue can be so clearly defined and evaluated. The Senate rules permit only "aye" and "nay" responses: votes of "maybe" are unacceptable.

A lifetime of academic training which had taught me not to act until all the data were in and I was sure of my conclusions was thus rudely and abruptly upended in the real world of Congress. Perhaps the most important lesson I learned from my experience there was that most issues cannot be expressed in black and white terms and that in the real world, those who are given responsibility to act for society can only make the best assumptions and reach the best conclusions available *at a particular time;* they must also act on that basis, and then hope for the best. I have emphasized this point here, not only because it was a great personal revelation for me but because this phenomenon is no less true in the federal executive bureaucracy than it is in the Congress, a point that should be kept in mind because of its importance to the story of swine flu.

My feeling of shock at the way Congress worked was matched by my feeling of surprise and disappointment at how little I was able to use my scientific skills while doing my job as a congressional staff man. While in a vague and general way I was charged by the staff director of the subcommittee with "keeping an eye" on biomedical affairs in general, and on the National Institutes of Health in particular, yet most of my specific assignments had little to do with science per se. Thus, I became deeply involved in staffing a bill sponsored jointly by Senator Kennedy and Senator Gary Hart of Colorado, aimed at forcing the tobacco industry to move faster toward a "safer" cigarette by imposing a stiff tax on its tar and nicotine content. Here, however, the question had less to do with the scientific data relating cigarette smoking to cancer and heart disease than with the interplay of political forces represented by the Tobacco Institute and the tobacco-state senators on the one side, and the American Cancer Society and Heart Association on the other. Also, I spent much time working with Eunice Shriver, Senator Kennedy's sister, on a bill to provide various health services to pregnant teenagers, and became something of an instant expert on the medical and sociological problems of pregnant young women and their offspring. But here too, the issue was less one of health legislation than of the highly charged politics involved in the fight between various pro- and anti-abortionist groups. Another issue on which I spent much time came under the general rubric of "international health" and centered on how to improve the efforts of the United States in helping the underdeveloped nations of the Third World prevent and treat the many tragic diseases with which they are afflicted. Once again, however, the problem had less to do with medical science than with medical and foreign politics, for it involved severe jurisdictional disputes among congressional committees and within the federal bureaucracy; unfortunately, the starving and diseased poor of Asia, Africa, and South America have no strong constituency in the United States to press their cause.

When, in March of 1976, the president announced the swine flu immunization program and sent the bill to Congress to be acted upon, I almost shouted aloud with relief and glee. Finally, after six months of drought, I would have a *real* scientific problem to deal with. More than that, it was a problem within my own area of expertise, since, as an immunologist, I was supposed to know something about immunizations — and in fact, I had done some laboratory work with the influenza virus itself during an earlier pandemic in 1957. My glee was short-lived, however, for I was quickly disabused of the notion that this was a question on which Science would triumph. As the months passed and Congress dealt with the swine flu issue in its various forms, it soon became apparent that the course of events was being decided more by political and occasionally economic considerations than by scientific ones. For the first time, I witnessed in great detail the sometimes subtle, sometimes not so subtle, influences that affect the course of events in government. The swine flu issue brought into play the frictions that exist between a Republican presidency and a Democratic Congress, the frictions and differences of style between the Senate and the House of Representatives, and the frictions between congressional committees vying to protect their own jurisdictional rights. Finally and not least, there were the political consequences of all of this happening in a presidential election year.

I should make it clear immediately that when I claim that "politics" entered into the consideration at different stages, I am not implying anything dirty or underhanded, for I also learned during my stay in the Senate no longer to use the word *politics* in a pejorative sense. Thus, when a Kennedy asks his staff man what the electorate in Massachusetts thinks about a certain issue, or when he bargains with the minority members of his subcommittee or with his counterpart in the House for support of a bill, or when the president considers the electorate or the Congress in deciding how to deal with an issue — these are all examples of "politics," but in its finest sense. They reflect not only a responsiveness to the will of the people (although this factor will not always be decisive in their decision of what is the best course to take) but also an understanding that politics is "the art of the possible" and that few bills are signed into law that have not involved some degree of concessions, trade-offs, and compromise.

I thus saw the swine flu issue unfold at first hand, as I staffed it on behalf of Senator Kennedy and the Senate Health Subcommittee. Even from the strictly congressional point of view, it was so complex and fascinating that I remember thinking at the time that it would make an interesting case study of the political process as it involves an important health issue. Inertia alone would probably have been sufficient to keep me from writing anything about swine flu when I returned to my laboratory after a year's stay in Congress, but something else very curious occurred that almost assured that I would do nothing about it. In spite of a certain sadness at leaving the center of power that is Washington and the U.S. Senate, and at quitting the frenetic hustle and bustle of hard work, quick decisions, and rapid action that I had not only become accustomed to but had even grown to like, the old serenity of my laboratory in Baltimore almost overwhelmed me on my return. For the first time in over a year I could put my feet on my desk and *think about what I was doing,* and carefully and methodically design future experiments in pursuit of my first love, immunology. There was no way that I would give up this now-revivified scientific passion to relive the swine flu experience — and besides, that was more a job for a political scientist than for a biomedical researcher.

The months rolled gently by, and I was only dimly aware that with the new Carter administration in place, the previous assistant secretary of health, Theodore Cooper, had been replaced; that the new secretary of HEW, Joseph Califano, had called the swine flu affair a fiasco and had fired as its chief culprit the head of the Center for Disease Control, David Sencer; and finally, that Califano had commissioned an outside study of this fiasco by Professors Richard Neustadt and Harvey Fineberg of Harvard University. Since almost two years would elapse between the swine flu episode and the Neustadt-Fineberg report, and since I was now once again ensconced in my academic ivory tower, I looked forward to reading the report, less to see if my ideas about it would be confirmed than from the now almost passive interest that one sometimes has in an event that took place in the distant past.

Although I started reading *The Swine Flu Affair: Decision-Making on a Slippery Disease* in an almost casual manner,[1] I hadn't got far into it before I found myself reading more intently, muttering to myself, "That's not what really happened," and "My God! They left out the fascinating part about . . ." By the time I had finished the volume, I found myself jolted out of my lethargy about swine flu and excited about the good old days of hyperactivity in the Senate. I felt that, somehow, Neustadt and Fineberg had gotten it all wrong. As I reflected on the matter, however, I decided that I had been too hasty in my conclusion. The swine flu report was not erroneous in describing *what* had happened, but I felt it was far off the mark in explaining *why* certain things had happened.

Neustadt and Fineberg concluded that "too much had been decided too early," and that the chief culprits in the matter were the "wily bureaucrat" David Sencer and his boss, Theodore Cooper, the two top government health officials involved. I, on the other hand, had the very strong impression that Sencer and Cooper had done nothing less than fulfill their assigned responsibilities to oversee the health of the American people, and that once swine flu had been detected in New Jersey in early 1976, events had unfolded inexorably like a Greek drama over which serious and competent government officials could exert little control. For me, the chief culprit in the case was swine flu itself, because it confounded the experts by not returning during the fall and winter of 1976. A secondary culprit was Legionnaires' Disease, which broke out in early August of 1976, for it revivified the federal immunization program which might have otherwise died. The final culprit was certainly the Guillain-Barré syndrome, which appeared in November and December of 1976, since the identification of this disease as a consequence of swine flu immunization caused the cancellation of the National Influenza Immunization Program and also assured that the entire venture would be marked as a fiasco.

My interest in swine flu was now not only revived, but intensified. Whereas previously I had only considered it to be an interesting case study in the political process, of primarily academic interest, now I felt that there was a more important reason to try to set the story straight. Not only had government health officials, and indirectly the entire scientific community, been erroneously indicted and convicted because of a lack of general understanding of both the nature of the influenza virus and of the true function of preventive medicine; but far worse, a misperception of what had happened in 1976 could cripple governmental efforts to cope with the next massive influenza pandemic, which will surely come sometime in the future. As we shall see, it is the peculiar nature of the influenza virus to change its structure, so that immunity to earlier forms of the virus does not necessarily protect against the new arrival — and history has shown that sooner or later a new strain will arise somewhere in the world and spread like wildfire in pandemic form. If the conclusion was accepted that the scientists and government health officials had over-reacted in 1976, and that some of their heads had rolled as a result, then the clear danger existed that when the next influenza pandemic arrived, public health officials, fearing for their jobs, might postpone action, at great cost in human disease and death.

In order to confirm my impressions of the Neustadt-Fineberg report and also to test my assumptions about what had really happened during the swine flu affair of 1976, I consulted four persons who had been intimately involved in the affair and whose opinions I respected highly. These were Leroy Goldman, Senator Kennedy's former staff director of the Senate Health Subcommittee; Jay Cutler, Senator Jacob Javits's former minority counsel on the Health Subcommittee; Stephen Lawton, staff director of Congressman Paul Rogers's Health Subcommittee in the House of Representatives; and Harold Schmeck, medical reporter of the *New York Times*. These four were unanimous in their conclusions: (1) that Neustadt and Fineberg had somehow misinterpreted much of what had occurred during the swine flu affair of 1976; (2) that they were in general agreement with the ideas that I had briefly outlined to them about what had happened and why; and (3) that I should try to set the record straight.

There was yet another reason why I consulted specifically with Lee Goldman. An informal rule, known to the staff of the Senate Health Subcommittee as Goldman's Commandment, stated: "Thou shalt not write about what thou hast seen or heard while working in this office." One of the conditions imposed upon me, when I was taken onto the staff of the Senate Health Subcommittee, was that I abide by this commandment. It had its origin in the occasional experience around the Senate that a staffer, and especially a short-term congressional fellow, would work for a time on a committee staff or in the office of a Member of the Senate, and then leave, to write an exposé of the personal and political foibles of Members of Congress or their staffs. People had been burned often enough in this manner, so that one analog or another of the Goldman Commandment was taken quite seriously throughout the Congress. If I were to write about swine flu, then I threatened to contravene the commandment, and therefore I felt obliged to appeal for an exemption from its strictures. When I explained my predicament to him, Goldman quickly granted me the exemption I sought, and my conscience rests easy in writing the report that follows.

In gathering material for this book, extensive use was made of my own files on the congressional involvement in the swine flu affair, as well as numerous original governmental documents and reports and the contemporary commentaries that appeared in both the scientific literature as well as the public press. I am deeply indebted to all of those people inside and outside the government who so generously made available to me so much of this material. I also personally interviewed most of the principal participants in this drama, and deeply appreciate the willingness of all of these individuals to reexamine with me this incident from the past, an incident which many of them would probably prefer to forget. I hope that I have done justice to them and to their ideas, and I apologize in advance to any who feel that their actions or thoughts have been misinterpreted. While this review of the swine flu affair is not intended to be a polemic on behalf of my own favored theses, it has proved impossible to avoid letting my biases show, and for this I make no apology.

This last caveat should especially be kept in mind by those readers in search of a "definitive history" of the swine flu affair. This report is not directed at the serious scholar, although references are given to most of the primary sources used. Rather, it is directed at the nonspecialist who is interested in the health sciences, or in politics, or who just wishes to understand the forces around him that affect his life. It will suffice if the reader finds the story interesting, and will succeed if the reader is stimulated to reflect upon the implications of the swine flu affair for the broad field of public policy decision-making, and for the narrower field of government involvement in public health and preventive medicine.

I must, finally, express my appreciation to those who made this report possible: to my wife, who put up with my prolonged absences during that year; to the Federation of American Societies for Experimental Biology for sponsoring my Congressional Fellowship year; to Senator Edward M. Kennedy and the staff of the Senate Health Subcommittee, for providing me with a marvelous education in the political and legislative processes; to those who read portions of or all of the text, for their helpful criticisms; to David Andrews, for his editing skills; and to Mrs. Irene Skop, for her efficient and tireless assistance with the manuscript.

CHAPTER 1

Swine Flu Strikes Again

I NFLUENZA is a curious disease. To the medical scientist, it is only the disease that results from infection with the influenza virus, accompanied by such symptoms as fever, headache, sore muscles, coughing or sneezing, and runny nose or watery eyes. For most of the rest of us, influenza is not a specific virus, but a nonspecific disease that makes us feel miserable for a few days and may even cause us to take to our beds for a time. We call it "flu," or "the grippe," or "the virus," and are usually content to make our own diagnoses and prescribe our own treatment, knowing that it probably will not be much worse this time than it was all the other times that we suffered from it. The symptoms are so nonspecific, and we are so used to seeing them appear each year when the weather turns cold, that we use the term flu indiscriminately to cover a wide variety of disease agents; we even talk about intestinal flu, although this common complaint has nothing to do with the influenza virus.

In most years it is difficult to know how much true influenza disease actually exists in the population, and for most of us it makes little difference. There are people, however, who are vitally concerned about influenza and who try to keep close track of its comings and goings. These are the doctors who work for large corporations or for school districts, for whom influenza may mean serious problems of absenteeism. These are also the federal, state, and local public health officers, whose duty it is to look out for the health of the people under their care. These experts know full well that while influenza is usually a mild disease, it may cause death in a small proportion of cases, usually among small children or elderly people. These experts know that even though the death rate may be only one in a thousand cases or less, in the years when influenza spreads widely through the population, the toll may be very great. Another group keenly interested in the influenza virus is the medical corps of the armed services. Doctors there know that influenza is one of the leading causes of absence from duty of soldiers and sailors. They have seen influenza put whole units of the army or navy out of action, and they are aware that influenza caused more deaths during the First World War than did enemy bullets.

1

Thus, both civilian and military public health experts wish to know as early as possible when *real* influenza is spreading, so that they can take action to prevent individual disease by immunization and also to prevent the spread of disease by closing schools or by limiting the movement of troops.

The winter of 1975–76 was a cold and dreary one in the northeastern United States, and seemed especially so in the flatlands of New Jersey around the army post at Fort Dix, where each year many thousands of fresh recruits are given their basic training. Shortly after the new year, a new contingent of recruits arrived, and with them came the typical assortment of upper respiratory diseases that the army expects to see when a large group of people is brought together from all over the country, exchanging novel bacteria and viruses with one another. The daily sick calls were well attended, and many soldiers were excused from duty, some even going to the hospital.

There had been an earlier outbreak of upper respiratory disease at Fort Meade, Maryland, from which specimens were sent to the virology laboratory at Walter Reed Army Medical Center in Washington, D.C. The outbreak was identified as due to an adenovirus, which is unrelated to influenza virus but which causes mild, flu-like symptoms. In view of the Fort Meade findings, Col. Joseph Bartley, the chief of preventive medicine at Fort Dix, presumed that his outbreak was also due to adenovirus and, following normal routine, reported these illnesses through army channels and also to the civilian health department in New Jersey. At the civilian health department the report came to the attention of Dr. Martin Goldfield, the assistant commissioner of the New Jersey Department of Public Health and its laboratory chief. Dr. Goldfield thought that the Fort Dix outbreak was more likely to be due to influenza virus rather than adenovirus, and he asked the army to send some specimens up to the New Jersey Public Health Laboratories for analysis. Goldfield had so much confidence in his hunch that he even made a small wager with Colonel Bartley on the outcome of the laboratory tests.

It is not difficult for a well-equipped virology laboratory to confirm the presence of influenza virus in a sick patient. Since influenza is an upper respiratory disease, a specimen can easily be obtained by taking a small washing from the nose or a swab of the throat. The suspected material is then inoculated into live embryonated chicken eggs and allowed to incubate for a few days; if the influenza virus is present, it will grow in the fluids of the chick embryo. The fluids are then tested for the presence of influenza virus by mixing them with washed red blood cells. If influenza virus is present, it will agglutinate, or clump, these cells, due to the presence of a special protein on the surface of the virus called a hemagglutinin. If the red cells do not clump together, then no influenza virus is present.

The technicians at the New Jersey laboratory worked on nineteen specimens in all from the Fort Dix outbreak, and in eleven obtained a positive test for influenza virus. While winning the wager for Dr. Goldfield, these findings meant that another step was needed in the laboratory procedure. In addition to knowing that the influenza virus is responsible for disease, the virologist also wants to know what strain of influenza virus is involved. Unlike most disease agents, influenza is curious because it can spontaneously change its surface molecules from time to time. Each such change means not only that a new strain of virus has appeared but also that any immunity which might have developed from exposure to earlier strains might be rendered useless, depending upon how different the new strain is from the old one. Again, it is not a very difficult task to identify influenza virus strains, since each virology laboratory will usually have special reagents on hand for all of the common strains of influenza virus which have been isolated in previous years.

It took only three or four days for the New Jersey lab not only to show that eleven of the nineteen Fort Dix specimens had influenza virus but also to confirm that most of these isolates contained the influenza strain that was then common throughout much of the world, called A/Victoria. What disturbed the virologists, however, was that they were completely unable to identify two of the virus isolates and were unsure about five others. While this in itself was not a very troubling or unusual finding, Goldfield felt that he should fill in the gap in the story by sending the seven suspect specimens for analysis by leading influenza virus experts. He therefore sent the specimens to the main federal laboratory at the Center for Disease Control (CDC) in Atlanta.

Not only is CDC charged with administering a variety of federal programs in preventive medicine and disease control, through extensive collaborations with state and local health officials, but it also furnishes important technical backup for public health officers and laboratories by providing the most up-to-date laboratory techniques, facilities, and reagents to assist in diagnostic problems. Additionally, CDC serves as the national center for disease surveillance and for the dissemination of information about disease problems. Among the different units at CDC is one that specializes in influenza, a laboratory whose competence is so widely recognized that it has been designated as a World Health Organization Influenza Reference Centre.

While the unidentified virus specimens were on their way by mail from the New Jersey health laboratory to the CDC laboratory in Atlanta, recruits at Fort Dix continued to report at sick call with flulike disease. On

February 4, 1976, Private David Lewis reported in ill and was sent to bed, but he apparently felt well enough to participate in the five-mile march scheduled for that night as part of the regular training program. During the course of the march, Private Lewis collapsed, and in a matter of hours died of what was diagnosed as pneumonia of possible influenza origin. Over the next few days, the New Jersey health laboratory, continuing its study of specimens from the sick recruits at Fort Dix, was unable to identify the strain of two further influenza-positive specimens, and also sent these to CDC for analysis. One of these specimens had been taken from the corpse of Private Lewis.

On the same day that the two new specimens arrived at the Bureau of Laboratories at CDC, preliminary tests showed that five of the original seven New Jersey virus isolates were the familiar A/Victoria strain, but the remaining two, while almost certainly influenza, represented a different virus type. Over the next week, the CDC virologists applied their full battery of testing procedures in an attempt to identify the new strain of influenza that had emerged from the Fort Dix epidemic. By February 12, it seemed clear that the new virus was very closely related to the swine flu influenza virus that had first been isolated in the early 1930s and was thought by most experts to have been responsible for the great influenza pandemic of 1918–19.

The discovery of any major new influenza strain causing disease in the population is usually considered serious, since these are often the harbingers of a subsequent epidemic of influenza.[2] The finding of a new swine flu strain spreading disease in the human population was considered doubly serious, since human-to-human spread of swine influenza had not been seen for over fifty years. The CDC laboratory chief thought that this finding was so important that he telephoned the director of CDC, Dr. David Sencer, to inform him about it that evening. Sencer, who doubles as the top preventive medicine expert in the United States Public Health Service, immediately recognized the significance of the finding and urged the laboratory people to reconfirm that it was indeed swine influenza virus in the Fort Dix isolates, and he ordered them to report the results on the following day. When, on February 13, the CDC scientists confirmed to Sencer that the influenza isolates were in fact of the swine type, he knew immediately that he had a potentially very serious problem on his hands and that he must act quickly. Sencer asked Dr. Walter Dowdle, CDC's chief virologist, to telephone some of the leading government health officials around the country to notify them of the discovery of swine influenza virus and to invite them to an emergency meeting in Atlanta on the next day. At this meeting, in addition to many of the senior staff and scientists at CDC, would be Cols. Philip Russell and Frank Top of the

Walter Reed Army Institute of Research in Washington, since this virus had originated at Fort Dix; New Jersey's Dr. Goldfield, since the outbreak had occurred in his bailiwick; Dr. Harry Meyer, Jr., Director of the Bureau of Biologics of the Food and Drug Administration, since his unit had the responsibility for the licensing of influenza vaccines; and Dr. John Seal, Scientific Director of the National Institute of Allergy and Infectious Diseases of the National Institutes of Health in Bethesda, Maryland, since his Institute had the prime responsibility for government-sponsored research on viruses and viral diseases. All of the members of this group recognized, with Sencer, the implications of this reappearance of swine influenza virus in the human population, and they dropped everything else to fly to Atlanta for the meeting.

In order to understand the consternation that these government scientists must have felt when they learned that the swine influenza virus was loose in the land, the reader must become familiar with two aspects of influenza as they were understood in February of 1976. The first has to do with the long history of influenza-the-disease, as it ebbed and flowed during the previous several centuries, in some years exacting a fearful toll in disease and death and in other years appearing either not at all or only in a very benign form. The second important factor involves influenza-the-virus, that strange agent of disease almost unique in its ability to change forms and go about in disguise to spread disease, so that its resemblance to familiar influenza strains could be detected only by subtle laboratory tests. Although remarkable strides had been made over the previous forty years, firm scientific knowledge about the epidemiologic history of the disease and about the molecular biology of the virus still left much to be desired. The science of influenza in 1976, therefore, was (and still is) somewhat impure.

Without an appreciation of both the history and the science of influenza, it will not be possible to understand why the swine flu affair of 1976 unfolded as it did.

CHAPTER 2

Influenza:
The Last Great Plague

THROUGHOUT recorded history, massive outbreaks of infectious diseases have periodically spread through the world, leaving great swaths of death and destruction in their wake. In some cases they were restricted to limited areas and are referred to as *epidemics,* while in other instances they would sweep like wildfire in *pandemic* form to afflict almost simultaneously much of the world's population. There are repeated descriptions of a variety of plagues and pestilences in the Old Testament and in the writings of most of the historians of early civilization, although in retrospect it is usually impossible to define the specific disease involved from the incomplete contemporary descriptions.[3] Only from medieval times onward can we begin to put specific names on these outbreaks of disease and feel some confidence in ascribing them to bubonic or pneumonic plague, smallpox, malaria, or yellow fever, and so on.

Each time one of these diseases spreads through a population, it inflicts a greater or lesser degree of sickness *(morbidity)* or death *(mortality),* depending upon the intrinsic virulence of the infectious agent and the susceptibility of the population at risk. Thus, true plague, caused by the bacterial agent *Pasteurella pestis* (named after the great bacteriologist Louis Pasteur), revisited the world periodically from at least the fifth century up to the early twentieth century and in its cruelest form, during the Black Plague of the fourteenth century, is estimated to have exterminated over one-third of the total population of Europe. Similar ravages occurred among the Aztec and Inca populations of the New World when the conquistadors brought smallpox with them, and among Eskimo populations in the north and native populations in the Pacific islands when they first encountered the measles virus. William McNeill, in his fascinating book, *Plagues and Peoples,*[4] not only describes the impressive mortality that accompanied these various epidemics and pandemics but also advances some imaginative speculations on how these diseases may have affected the course of history.

Decade after decade and century after century, the great killers came and went with no detectable regularity, and there was little that could be done about them. Neither the agents of these diseases nor their modes of transmission were understood. While some speculated during the sixteenth and seventeenth centuries that "seeds" or "germs" might cause disease, these were little more than words to express the unknown or even unknowable. Indeed, when Anton van Leeuwenhoek perfected his microscope and described little "animalcules" in dirty water and on food, he did not dream of associating them with disease agents. Even after bacteria were carefully described and connected with disease, many people refused to believe that the relationship was a specific one. Bacteria (like flies, worms, and even mice) were thought by serious scientists to arise by a spontaneous generation from filth and muck,[5] and it was not until the 1870s and 1880s that Louis Pasteur and Robert Koch were able to convince many of them otherwise.

Even the origin of these deadly diseases was clouded in mystery. While earlier cultures had been content to view disease as an individual or collective punishment for sin or transgression, delivered by the arrows of a Phoebus Apollo or cast among the people by a wrathful God, the more rational period of the Renaissance saw other theories advanced. Some thought that epidemics of disease were the result of unfavorable conjunctions of the stars, while others, harking back to ancient Greek ideas, agreed that disease must originate from airborne miasmas, and found in the ill winds and waters of a locality the source of their problems, with sickness arising from bad air *(mal-aria)*. This latter theory held sway for a surprisingly long time. Even into the late nineteenth century and the early years of the present century, many reputable scientists and public health officials refused to acknowledge that such diseases as influenza and cholera might be contagious; the rapidity of their spread in a country or throughout the world appeared to argue against person-to-person transmission.[6]

In the absence of information on the nature of these diseases, little could be done to prevent their spread or to aid in their cure. In some places, ships were quarantined as early as the fifteenth century, but with the ever-increasing growth of trade and the movement of peoples, this became less and less adequate as a measure of prevention. In individual cases, the wealthy might flee in the face of epidemic disease, as the characters in Boccaccio's *Decameron* did, but this escape was available to only a few. And finally, when disease actually arrived, the armamentarium of the physician permitted little more than the treatment of individual symptoms, and for centuries the usual practice of purging and bleeding and applying leeches to the patient probably did more harm than good.

During these centuries, until the development of a scientific bacteriology and theories of public health, only one infectious disease proved amenable to *preventive* measures — smallpox. In many parts of the world, and apparently independently of one another, the folk practice developed of inoculating material from the pustules of active smallpox cases into healthy individuals, in order to give them a mild form of the disease and render them immune to the more disfiguring or deadly natural disease.[7] Voltaire thought, probably erroneously, that the practice had developed among the Circassians, who made it a custom to sell their daughters into Turkish harems and wished to prevent the smallpox scars that would inevitably lower the value of their commodity. Whatever its origins, the practice was well known in Constantinople at the beginning of the eighteenth century and was introduced into the Western world by the letters of two Greek physicians, Timoni and Pylarini, and by the example of Lady Mary Wortley Montagu, wife of the British ambassador to the Sultan's court, who had her children inoculated. Where it was accepted, inoculation did much good in preventing smallpox, but it was superseded by the much safer and more effective vaccination procedure introduced in 1796 by Edward Jenner. This immunization procedure was so effective that it not only sharply reduced the incidence of smallpox infection over the next 150 years but also provided the mechanism for the final and total eradication of this disease, following a thirteen-year campaign by the World Health Organization (WHO), which finally ended successfully in 1979.[8]

But if smallpox could be dealt with so effectively and this early, the other great killer diseases had to await the golden age of bacteriology, from about 1880 to 1910, for the isolation of their specific agents and the demonstrations by Louis Pasteur and others of how to use these agents for preventive immunization. As each of these agents was isolated and its mode of transmission identified, methods were devised to deal with them. In some cases, as with plague, diphtheria, and tetanus, simple immunization procedures sufficed. In other cases, such as cholera, immunization proved relatively ineffective, but an understanding that the organism spread through contaminated water meant that adequate public health sanitation measures might prove effective against the disease. In yet other instances, such as yellow fever, the demonstration by Walter Reed in Cuba that the agent is transmitted by the mosquito made possible, through mosquito eradication campaigns, the construction of the Panama Canal.

Thus, even though preventive measures are not always utilized or feasible (cholera is still a significant disease in Southeast Asia, and malaria in Africa and elsewhere), at least the theoretical basis for a preventive medicine exists for these diseases.

One by one, the worldwide killer diseases have been banished, or at least neutralized and restricted to increasingly more limited areas of the world, with the expectation that sooner or later they will be abolished as serious threats to humanity. In the early days of the microbiologic era, the most effective campaigns to eliminate disease were waged against those illnesses caused by bacterial organisms that were large enough to be seen in the light microscope. As time went on, it became apparent that some diseases were caused by organisms that were too small to be seen in a microscope, organisms that would pass through the finest filter. These were called ultrafilterable viruses, and with the development of techniques to isolate and grow them in chick embryos or in tissue culture and to see them with the electron microscope, the virologist and immunologist have learned to cope with viral diseases also. Over the years, effective vaccines have been developed against yellow fever, poliomyelitis, measles, mumps, German measles, and others, so that mankind no longer need be subjected to repeated epidemics of these diseases.

Influenza

Medical science has thus, in the last century, developed the capability of ridding the world once and for all of the ravages of most epidemic and pandemic infectious diseases. Medical students in advanced nations that are able to utilize all of these techniques scarcely know how to diagnose a case of smallpox, or of whooping cough, and will soon have only textbooks to consult for descriptions of some of the infectious diseases that only recently affected us or our children. There is one disease, however, that medical students will probably continue to see now and in the future, just as succeeding generations have seen it in the past. This disease is influenza, which W. I. B. Beveridge has called "the last great plague,"[9] because it is the last of the great infectious agents that trouble mankind for which biomedical research has not been able to propose even a theoretically permanent solution.

It is not clear when influenza was first recognized as a separate disease entity, although it did get its name during the fifteenth century when some sort of upper respiratory disease was ascribed to the influence (Italian: *influenza*) of the stars. Epidemics of influenza were certainly known during the Elizabethan period, although insofar as we can tell from early descriptions, these were often more discommoding than life-threatening. Thus, it was reported by Lord Randolph from the court of Mary, Queen of Scots, in a letter to Lord Cecil in November, 1562:

> Maye it please your Honor, immediately upon the Quene's arivall here, she fell acquainted with a new disease that is common in this towne,

called here the newe acquayntance, which passed also throughe her whole courte, neither sparinge lordes, ladies nor damoysells not so much as ether Frenche or English. It ys a plague in their heades that have yt, and a sorenes in their stomackes, with a great coughe, that remayneth with some longer, with others shorter tyme, as yt findeth apte bodies for the nature of the disease. The queen kept her bed six days. There was no appearance of danger, nor manie that die of the disease, excepte some olde folkes. My lord of Murraye is now presently in it, the lord of Lidlington hathe had it, and I am ashamed to say that I have byne free of it, seinge it seketh acquayntance at all men's handes.[10]

As I noted above, influenza, unlike many epidemic diseases, is almost always present somewhere in the community. In off-years it may not be remarked, being readily confused with the common cold and a wide variety of other mild complaints. But it is unmistakable when it appears in epidemic form, as it does much more often than was true of other serious infectious diseases in their heyday. Shortly after the American Revolution, Noah Webster described influenza as an "epidemic and pestilential disease," and reported (on very questionable evidence) that there had been some forty-four appearances since the year 1174. He believed, with most medical experts of the time, that "the causes most probably exist in the elements fire, air, and water, for we know of no other medium by which diseases can be communicated to whole communities of people," and concluded that influenza is "evidently the effect of some insensible qualities of the atmosphere."[11]

Throughout the Middle Ages, there were numerous reports of epidemic disease that might have been influenza, and a true pandemic probably occurred in 1510. It was said to have come from Africa, and while it spread throughout Europe with a very high attack rate, it was accompanied by few deaths. However, in 1580, what was possibly the first truly global outbreak of influenza on record occurred. It was reported to have started in Asia, and spread rapidly throughout Africa, Europe, and America, and it was so virulent that within a period of six weeks it had raced through all of the nations of Europe, affecting so many people that those who were spared became objects of wonder to their neighbors. Of special interest — since it is so typical of modern influenza pandemics — reports from Britain indicated that two waves of disease were seen, one in the summer and one in the autumn. The pandemic of 1580 was also more virulent, and some nine thousand persons were reported to have died of it in Rome alone. Again, reports from that period mention that "all conditions of persons were attacked . . . those who were very strong and hardy were taken in the same manner as the weak and spoiled . . . the youngest as well as the oldest."[12] This age-independent attack rate is also typical of modern influenza.

The Incidence of Influenza Pandemics

Since the historical record makes it clear that pandemics of influenza have occurred at intervals for a very long time, it is important to know the frequency of these onslaughts. Beveridge has attempted such a historical analysis, but he points out that the records that exist prior to the eighteenth century are too vague and irregular to permit a satisfactory analysis. However, records improved after the year 1700, and Beveridge was able to assemble a tentative list by examining the reports from many countries. We must observe his cautionary note that a good deal of arbitrary judgment was necessary because of incomplete records and because changes in total population and in the extent and rapidity of human movement might have made epidemics behave differently in different centuries; yet his information points up several interesting facts.

Figure 1 presents Beveridge's findings on the occurrence of pandemics over the past 250 years. Some of these, represented by the long lines, could definitely be established as having been of world-wide incidence, while others (the short lines), more difficult to assess, were thus termed "possible" pandemics. It is apparent from the chart that these outbreaks of influenza occurred at quite irregular intervals. If all twenty of these outbreaks are considered to have been major pandemics, then their intervals varied from three to twenty-eight years, with an average of about twelve years between major incursions of the disease. If we accept only the ten outbreaks that Beveridge feels were unquestionably pandemics, then the intervals vary from ten to forty-nine years, with an average world-wide pandemic interval of some twenty-four years. This means not only that influenza has been with us for a very long time but that it continues, even in this modern era of high technology medicine and of vaccines and other efficacious tools of preventive medicine.

It has been suggested that major pandemics of the disease may occur at roughly eleven year intervals from now on.[13] Accepting the 1946 outbreak as a true pandemic, the intervals between the last three events (1946, 1957, 1968) have been exactly eleven years. The proposal was made that the interval between major pandemics may have decreased since the Second World War, owing to the recent vast increase in the amount of intercontinental travel, which may promote the more rapid dissemination of the virus. As we shall see below, this is consistent with the notion that new pandemics stem from changes in the virus itself and that the introduction of a new virus strain may be fostered by the development in the population of increasing levels of immunity to the old strain. Thus, the sooner we all are infected by the current strain and develop immunity to it, the more readily it may give way to a new pandemic strain.

THE INFLUENZA CHRONICLE

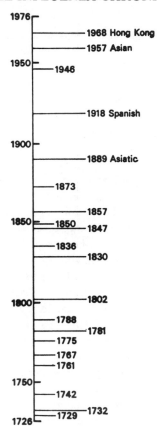

Figure 1. Pandemics during the last 250 years. The long lines represent ten definite pandemics, the shorter lines ten possible pandemics. Between the pandemics there were many "ordinary" epidemics that are not shown. (Reprinted with permission from W.I.B. Beveridge, *Influenza, The Last Great Plague* [New York: Prodist, 1977].)

It is interesting, as Beveridge and others point out, that so many of the influenza pandemics appear to have originated in Asia. As long ago as 1928, in his book *The Genesis of Epidemics,* Clifford Gill noted that "all authorities are agreed that pandemics of influenza can almost invariably be traced to 'the silent spaces' of Asia, Siberia, and Western China." [14] It is with good reason that in modern times so many of these outbreaks have been called Asiatic flu or Russian flu or Hong Kong flu. But what is most interesting for this story is that the great epidemic of 1918–19, although it was known throughout the world as Spanish influenza, did not originate in Spain. Even in its initial wave, it spread so rapidly that it is difficult to ascertain where, in fact, the first cases occurred. Epidemiologic detectives seem to have narrowed down the birthplace of Spanish influenza to two possible locations: the classical breeding ground of influenza in Western China and, most improbably, Fort Riley, Kansas.

The Epidemiology of Influenza

Influenza, as I have indicated, is a highly contagious disease. After the virus reponsible for it was isolated in the 1930s, it was quickly appreciated how much of the virus can be found early after infection, not only in the nose and throat but also in the tiny droplets that are sneezed out or coughed and spit up. It was easy to see how it could spread so rapidly, especially in close and crowded places like schools, vehicles, and army camps.

Influenza, as we have seen, is almost always present in the population. In some years it affects only a small number of people and in other years may spread like wildfire and touch almost everyone. In most years, the disease itself is usually benign, resulting in little more than annoying aches and sniffles, and perhaps a few days in bed. At these times, the principal complications are generally experienced only by very young children and by the elderly and infirm, who may get a complicating and potentially fatal viral or bacterial pneumonia. This is a well-known phenomenon to health statisticians, who usually lump these fatalities under the single title "Influenza and Pneumonia Deaths." They measure the severity of an epidemic in terms of *excess deaths,* that is, the number of deaths in any given period over and above those that would have been expected, based on previous experience over the course of many nonepidemic years.

In certain years, the influenza virus appears to change its habits, for reasons that are not understood by scientists. The virus may spread more efficiently, the *attack rate* (the proportion of the population that becomes ill) may increase dramatically, or the virulence of the virus may unaccountably increase, so that the disease in any individual may be more severe, and the proportion of deaths greater. In addition, this disease, which is usually serious only for the very young, the very old, and the very ill, sometimes unaccountably spares these high-risk groups and, instead, exacts its toll from among strong, healthy young adults.

Two other factors are important in understanding the epidemiology of influenza. First, when a new strain of influenza virus appears somewhere in the world, it may not spread immediately in pandemic form. Instead, it

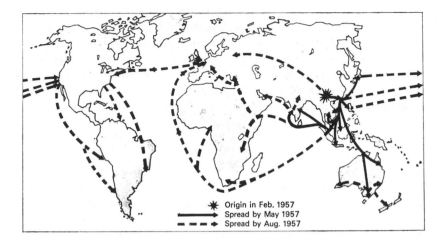

Figure 2. The spread of Asian influenza around the world. It started in China in February 1957. (Reprinted with permission from Beveridge, *Influenza: The Last Great Plague.*)

may affect a small number of people, go into hiding for a while, then appear elsewhere in sporadic outbreaks, and thus only slowly gain momentum until it emerges in its full epidemic force. The reasons for this are not at all well understood. Scientists suspect that it may have something to do with a phenomenon known as "adaptation to the host." It is a common laboratory finding that when an agent that causes disease in one species is used to infect another species, it may not grow well or cause disease until it has been passed many times from one host to another, with infectivity and virulence often increasing with each passage. Adaptation of a new flu virus to the human may take on special significance if, as discussed below, these new strains really arise from animal reservoirs.

Equally mysterious is the second important fact about the influenza virus. When a new strain of the virus spreads, any earlier strain still present in the population appears to submerge and disappear as a source of disease. It is as though the two strains occupy the same small ecological niche, with the new strain enjoying a competitive advantage over the old strain and forcing it into some sort of Darwinian extinction.

Once the flu virus is "ready," it is able to spread around a country or the world with truly impressive speed, and in this age of high-speed travel, the term *jet-spread* aptly describes influenza's velocity. As an example, the maps in figures 2 and 3 show how pandemic influenza spread around the world during 1957. The new "Asian" virus seems to have originated somewhere in China during February 1957. It reached Hong Kong in April and, by May, had spread throughout Southeast Asia and to India

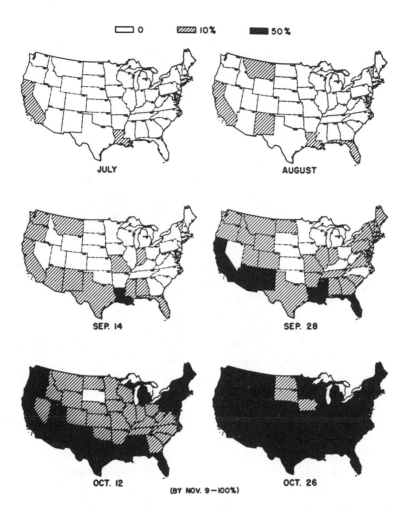

Figure 3. Progressive seeding of the United States with Asian (H2N2) influenza virus in summer-fall of 1957. Percentage of counties reporting influenza outbreaks, July-October 1957. (Reprinted with permission from Y. Trotter; F. L. Dunn; R. H. Drachman; D. A. Henderson; M. Pizzi; and A. D. Langmuir, "Asian Influenza in the United States, 1957–1958," *American Journal of Hygiene* 70 [1959]: 34.)

and Australia (solid lines on the map, figure 2). It then required less than three months to complete its spread over the entire world, and the pandemic was on. Figure 3 shows the rapid movement of Asian influenza in the United States during the summer and early autumn of 1957. It was first detected in July as isolated outbreaks in California and Louisiana (both important entry points to the United States). By August, it had spread slowly to four additional states, but it did not move rapidly until the first half of September, when it was reported in fourteen states. At that point, its spread accelerated, and in only six weeks had been reported in every state in the Union.

The Killer Flu of 1918–19

As the First World War dragged on into its fourth year across the battlefields of Europe, casualties continued to mount. This involved not only direct and indirect battlefield casualties among the military forces on both sides but also the inevitable casualties of hunger and disease that affect civilian populations as the consequence of widespread battle, the concentration and movement of large numbers of people, and the disruptions of normal patterns of existence. The cost of this war in terms of pain and suffering was fearsome, but paled in comparison with the return of pandemic influenza in the spring of 1918. The three successive waves of this disease that circled the world during the succeeding twelve months constituted the single greatest debacle that mankind has experienced in modern times and, second only to the Black Death, perhaps during all its history. By conservative estimates, the death toll throughout the world has been put at between 15 and 25 million human beings during that fateful year, a number not exceeded by all of the casualties of all of the wars of the twentieth century taken together. The agent responsible for this massive destruction of human life was later to be identified as swine influenza virus.

Contemporary accounts of that pandemic tell a story difficult to comprehend.[15] In many places more than half of the population was ill during a single influenza wave, resulting in the closing of schools and factories and in an almost complete breakdown in the normal patterns of life. Hospitals overflowed with the dead and dying, and in many places filled caskets were stacked like cordwood until they could be disposed of. The total mortality caused in the United States by the three waves of influenza was over 0.5 percent of the total population — more than 600,000 deaths. In England and Wales, the official figure was 200,000 deaths, and the mortality rate was on the same order in most Western countries. Elsewhere, the mortality rate was often much higher: in Alaska, some Eskimo villages were completely wiped out, and in Samoa one quarter of the entire population died. In India alone, it is estimated that 5 million people died, and in some cities the burial grounds and even the streets were, literally, covered with the dead.

In addition to these sobering mortality statistics, several other facets of the Spanish influenza pandemic are important for our story. The first is that many of the deaths associated with influenza infection were due to an accompanying bacterial pneumonia — this was an age when modern anti-biotics were not yet available. For a long time, in fact, medical men thought that influenza itself was due to Pfeiffer's bacillus (named after the German pathologist who discovered it in 1892), and this organism was given the scientific name *Hemophilus influenzae*. Only after the influenza virus had been isolated, in the 1930s, was it appreciated that all of the respiratory complaints, and some of the pneumonia cases, were caused by this virus, and that the viral disease might set the stage for complicating bacterial lung infection.

Second, like many other influenza epidemics and pandemics, the 1918 incident began with a relatively mild wave in the spring of 1918, accom-panied by a mortality rate that was not unusually high. That autumn, however, a second wave of the same disease appeared, a wave almost unparalleled in its lethal effects, and accounting for the greater proportion of the deaths ascribed to Spanish influenza. Finally, a third wave occurred early in 1919 which, while appreciably less severe than the second, also contributed significantly to both morbidity and mortality.

The third important aspect of this influenza pandemic involved the incidence of death among different age groups. I have already indicated that the high-risk groups in a typical influenza outbreak are the very young and the very old, and in this respect the first wave of Spanish influenza was fairly typical. But the second wave of influenza in 1918 was different. The death rate among children and the aged was not great, and death seemed selectively to choose the strongest and most healthy — those between 18 and 40 years old. Fully half of all deaths were in this age group, a finding that is almost unique in the modern history of influenza. Just how extraordinary this second wave of influenza was can be graphically seen in figure 4, where the age-specific death rate for Spanish influenza is compared with what we might call a "typical" influenza year. The differences are so striking that they can be seen at a glance.

Fourth, finally, when Spanish Influenza first appeared in the spring of 1918, the attack rate was found to vary with age in a curious manner. Fully 30 to 40 percent of all people under 35 years of age became ill, while only 20 percent of 50-year-olds and 10 percent of 70-year-olds showed clinical infection. It was almost as though the older age groups had had previous experience with the same virus, resulting in immunity that pro-tected them from the infection now raging. If this assumption was true, it would imply that this particular virus had occurred not only in 1918 but had appeared on the scene many years before, leaving the elderly of 1918 with some degree of immunity, but the young defenseless.

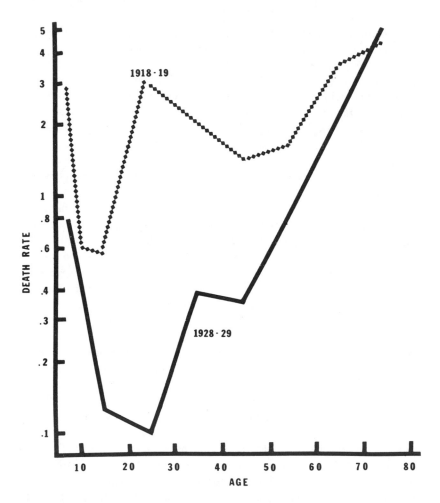

Figure 4. Death rate by age per 1,000 cases of influenza. A typical influenza year is characterized by a U-shaped curve, in which young adults are generally spared. In the 1918–19 pandemic, the line is W-shaped, indicating an abnormal mortality in the 20- to 40-year-age group.

Pandemics during the Modern Era

Three major outbreaks of influenza have occurred during the past thirty years, all widespread, but nowhere approaching the disastrous proportions of the Spanish influenza of 1918. In 1946, there was an outbreak of influenza which is usually classified as a mild pandemic, followed in 1957 by a severe pandemic, and in 1968 by a moderate pandemic. This

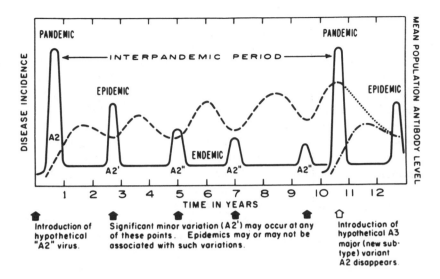

Figure 5. The hypothetical 11-year cycle of influenza pandemics. The solid line indicates the incidence of clinical disease, while the broken line shows the slowly increasing immunity in the population to the old strain of virus, which is rendered useless when the new pandemic strain appears. A2', A2", etc, represent successive variants of the original A2 strain of virus. (Reprinted with permission from Edwin D. Kilbourne, ed., *The Influenza Viruses and Influenza* [New York: Academic Press, 1975].)

eleven-year interval between recent outbreaks prompted Kilbourne to suggest that influenza might be settling down to a regular cycle,[16] as illustrated in figure 5. He suggests that a major pandemic might be expected periodically, followed by sporadic outbreaks of diminishing intensity during the interpandemic period, until a new virus strain arrives to start the cycle anew. Kilbourne's speculation was widely known in virologic and public health circles and was taken very seriously in 1976, since it not only seemed to explain the influenza picture of the previous thirty years but also to fit with the most recent information on the biology of the influenza virus.

It is estimated that the pandemic of 1957 cost the United States 70,000 excess deaths.[17] In addition, the total economic cost to our society in terms of death and disease, of health care cost, and of productive time lost was estimated at over $4 billion. Similarly, the milder pandemic of 1968 is thought to have cost the United States about 34,000 lives and some $2 to $3 billion. These figures are important, since they were used in the equation to calculate the potential cost-benefit relationships of the swine flu immunization program of 1976.

By the time of the 1957 outbreak, some progress had been made on the development of preventive vaccines against the influenza virus. While research on these vaccines was performed primarily in university virology laboratories, the vaccines were produced by some half-dozen pharmaceutical companies in the private sector and then distributed in part to the military, who employed the vaccine extensively, and in part to the civilian population through the regular, predominantly nongovernmental health care system. Recommendations regarding the composition of the influenza vaccines were made for the military by the Commission on Influenza of the Armed Forces Epidemiologic Board, and for the civilian sector by the Center for Disease Control and the Bureau of Biologics, with the advice of their civilian advisory committees. After the vaccines had been produced by the pharmaceutical manufacturers, it was the responsibility of the Bureau of Biologics to pass on their safety and efficacy prior to granting licenses for their use, as prescribed by federal law.

In the normal course, influenza vaccine was used in the civilian population only on a very restricted basis for high-risk groups, including the elderly and others with illnesses that might make them more susceptible to the complications of influenza. During the typical year, some 15 to 20 million doses of influenza vaccine were normally produced, of which 8 to 12 million might be employed in the civilian population. Although the vaccines were considered to be only 50 to 70 percent effective, they were widely credited with saving many lives among the high-risk group and with reducing the severity of disease when it did appear in the vaccinated individual. In addition, the flu vaccine was considered very safe to use. Apart from such occasional side effects as fever and sore muscles, serious complications were rare. Of some 100 million doses administered during the seven to eight years prior to 1976, only fifteen lawsuits had resulted, and all settlements had been modest.

In both 1957 and 1968, the first wave of the impending pandemic was detected some months before it struck the United States, because by then a world-wide surveillance system was in the process of organization, involving public health workers and laboratories in many parts of the world. On both occasions, public health officials in the United States took note of these outbreaks, and serious discussions were held about what might be done to limit the disease and its destructive consequences. In both instances, the exercise proved extremely frustrating for the public health officials involved.

When, in the spring of 1957, the first news arrived from Hong Kong that a new strain of influenza threatened, it appeared that there might be time to head off the danger. Throughout that spring and summer, the different scientific advisory committees kept close track of the situation, and they urged the production and distribution of massive amounts of the appropriate influenza vaccine.[18] They recommended, moreover, that the vaccine not be restricted only to high-risk cases but be disseminated as widely as possible throughout the American population, in order to diminish the personal and economic disruptions that invariably accompany influenza pandemics. The question was repeatedly raised whether the government itself should become involved in the immunization program, since past experience had demonstrated that distribution of vaccine through the private health care sector was not only less efficient, but was usually characterized by gross inequities of distribution. But the time did not seem socially ripe for such large-scale governmental involvement. The experts, fairly well attuned to the politics of the day probably, correctly concluded that Congress would be loathe to fund such a venture, and that it would inevitably be harmed by widespread cries of "socialized medicine." It was therefore decided that government agencies should restrict themselves, on the one hand, to urging the manufacturers to produce vaccine and on the other, to attempting to educate the public about the influenza threat, which would include recommending that people seek the vaccine through their usual channels.

As the influenza season of 1957 approached, vaccine production and public education both shifted into high gear, and when the expected outbreak of flu actually appeared in the United States, it seemed possible, for the first time in history, that the system might be ready to cope with the challenge. Sadly, these rosy expectations were deceived when the system broke down disastrously.

One cause of the breakdown was that there was almost never enough vaccine available in the right place at the right time. The pharmaceutical manufacturers had been asked to invest large amounts of money in vaccine, with no assurance that the pandemic would come and that they would be able to sell all of the vaccine they had produced. In many previous years, they had actually lost money on the fairly unprofitable vaccines, when many millions of doses were returned to them unused. Thus, while the vaccine producers did exert a reasonable effort to meet their public service obligation in the production of vaccine, they were understandably unwilling to commit themselves fully until the emergency actually arrived. By then, it was too late, since Asian influenza spread throughout the country in a matter of weeks. Anguished cries for vaccine from all over the United States could not be satisfied by the limited supplies available when the disease struck, although after the epidemic had run its course, tens of millions of doses of vaccine remained unused.

Another factor that contributed to the problem was the lack of preparedness by the health care system to deliver into the arms of the public those doses that were available. As experience with the administration of the Sabin live polio vaccine had shown many years before, an immense organizational effort is required to prepare vaccination centers, to mobilize doctors, nurses, and other volunteers to administer the injections, and to establish the pipeline that will assure delivery of the right amount of vaccine to the right place at the right time. In all of these respects, the immunization campaign of 1957 fell far short of the mark, and outraged complaints were voiced both by the public and by professionals.

The most outraged complaints in 1957 had to do with the inequities that accompanied the distribution of influenza vaccine through the private health care system. Some cities and states complained bitterly that their citizens had no vaccine, while other cities or states enjoyed adequate amounts. Far worse was the ability of some groups to bid successfully (on what was almost a black market) for vaccine that others could not afford. Cries of anguish arose when it was learned that certain large corporations had obtained all of the vaccine that they required to immunize their workers and keep their production lines going, while the poor and under-privileged in the inner cities could not obtain protection. Reports also appeared in the newspapers contrasting the ability of, for example, a baseball club to acquire enough vaccine to immunize its healthy players, while children and the high-risk elderly went without.

The situation in 1968 proved to be no better than it had been in 1957. The inefficiencies and inequities of these immunization programs not only angered the public but also left their mark upon the influenza scientists and public health officials — a memory that was to contribute importantly to the sequence of events in 1976.

The Message of Influenza History

It has been said that those who do not know history are destined to repeat it, and influenza scientists were by now well acquainted with the long history of influenza. They knew, during those early months of 1976, the following facts about influenza, summarized from the discussion above:

1. Influenza is never absent for very long in the population. For at least 250 years it returned *at unpredictable intervals,* in epidemic or pandemic form, to inflict great ravages on the people of the United States and of the entire world.

2. The most recent experience with influenza pandemics suggests that they may be coming with greater frequency, and an approximately

eleven-year pandemic cycle might now be established. *Thus, in 1976, a new pandemic might not be far off.*

3. *Virologic science had no way to predict in advance the severity of a pandemic.* Some pandemics are comparatively mild and are accompanied by few excess deaths, while others, like the Spanish influenza of 1918, killed on a scale rarely seen by mankind. Even a modest pandemic such as that in 1957 or 1968 might cause tens of thousands of deaths and many billions of dollars of economic damage.

4. *The lethal pandemic of 1918 was caused by a swine virus.* This virus had not been seen in the human population for over forty-five years, except for an occasional case in a person exposed to pigs: human-to-human transmission of swine influenza had not been seen since the early 1920s.

5. *Vaccines against influenza virus infection were available.* While these varied in their efficacy from about 50 to 80 percent effective, prior experience with several hundred million doses of influenza vaccine showed: (a) that they helped reduce morbidity and mortality; (b) that where they did not fully protect against disease, they often reduced its severity; and (c) that they were reasonably safe to use, with untoward side effects usually being limited to transient fever and muscle ache.

6. *Influenza pandemics spread like wildfire in this age of jet travel.* Therefore, any attempt to apply preventive vaccination to head off a pandemic imposed very tight time constraints on decision-making, planning, production, distribution, and administration of vaccine.

7. The pandemics of 1957 and 1968 showed that *voluntary immunization programs controlled and operated entirely through the private health sector were at best grossly inadequate and at worst near disasters.* The feeling had been growing that only the federal government could command the resources and impose the guidelines that would be required to mount so massive a venture in preventive medicine.

CHAPTER 3

Making Public Policy: Scientific Recommendations

E VERYONE who attended David Sencer's emergency meeting at the Center for Disease Control in Atlanta on February 14 was a professional in the public health field. They all had jobs that made them responsible, in one way or another, for the health of large numbers of people, and much of their normal activity was concerned with the prevention of infectious diseases. Sencer's CDC was the lead government agency in the detection and prevention of disease; John Seal's National Institute of Allergy and Infectious Diseases (NIAID) in Washington was responsible for the basic research on how infectious diseases develop and how they may be better treated or prevented; Harry Meyer's Bureau of Biologics (BoB) was responsible for quality control and the licensing of drugs and vaccines. Colonels Russell and Top of the army were responsible for the health of millions in the military, and Martin Goldfield's New Jersey Department of Health was charged with protecting the health of the citizens of his state. While none of them was an expert specifically in influenza, they all had seen epidemics of the disease during their medical careers and had seen people die of pneumonia as a result. They also knew, in very general terms, what influenza had inflicted in the past on the people of the world, and what they did not know specifically they would soon learn from the influenza experts on the CDC staff. Thus, with advance notice that swine flu had surfaced at Fort Dix, those who attended the emergency meeting must have gone in hoping for the best, but expecting the worst.

Sencer opened the meeting at 11:00 a.m. that Saturday by stressing the scientific aspects of the influenza outbreak at Fort Dix, rather than its pandemic disease implications. He then called upon CDC's chief virologist, Dr. Walter Dowdle, to review first the recent history of swine influenza and then the laboratory studies that positively identified some of the Fort Dix isolates as belonging to this strain of influenza virus. The question was raised, almost hopefully, whether the swine flu isolate might not represent a laboratory contaminant rather than a true finding — always a potential problem in any virology laboratory. While

24

Goldfield's laboratory in New Jersey did not have swine flu virus on hand, the CDC laboratory did. Therefore, the first order of business was to test new specimens that Goldfield had brought with him, using a "clean" laboratory in which no influenza work had ever been done. This would not only rule out laboratory contamination but would also provide yet another confirmation that the Fort Dix virus was indeed related to swine flu. In addition to this, the committee concentrated on the other types of information that would be required to confirm the severity and extent of the Fort Dix outbreak. The army promised to obtain additional specimens from the original sick soldiers and to take bleedings from large numbers of other Fort Dix trainees and from army dependents, in search of further evidence of spread of the virus. On its part, the New Jersey Department of Public Health prepared to begin an extensive surveillance of the civilian population around the Fort Dix area, to see whether the virus had spread beyond the bounds of the army camp.

Amid all of this low-key scientific discussion, it was inevitable that some mention was made of the possibility that the Fort Dix outbreak might mean that an influenza pandemic was in the offing. But while this issue was discussed, there was a marked tendency to underplay and postpone it, as though the very mention might bring the reality closer. Nevertheless, this idea was clearly in the minds of most of the participants, and it guided a number of the decisions made that day. Not only was further confirmation of the identity of the swine flu isolates and the follow-up search for additional infections in New Jersey to be accomplished as expeditiously as possible, but decisions were also made that appeared to anticipate an impending emergency. Thus, it was agreed that large amounts of specific antibody to the swine flu virus would be prepared, to assist in large-scale diagnostic procedures; large quantities of swine flu seed virus would be prepared, for possible distribution to influenza laboratories and to vaccine manufacturers around the country; and CDC agreed to commence work on the preparation of the special strains of swine flu virus that would be needed for high-yield egg culture, in the event that a massive vaccination program was undertaken. Indeed, in anticipation of this latter point, Goldfield had already sent specimens of the Fort Dix swine flu virus to Dr. Edwin Kilbourne of the Mount Sinai Medical School in New York; Kilbourne, one of the country's leading influenza experts, had pioneered in the development of techniques to increase the yield of viruses grown for vaccine. In addition, John Seal volunteered that NIAID would contact all the contractors engaged in its influenza work, in order to set up a special search for the swine flu virus elsewhere in the country, and Harry Meyer indicated that the Bureau of Biologics would send the high-yield strains of swine flu virus to the vaccine manufacturers as soon as they were available, so that early experience could be gained in their growth characteristics.

It was agreed that all of these actions should be completed as rapidly as possible, since even at that point it was understood by everyone involved that if the Fort Dix findings did indeed mean that a pandemic of influenza was on its way, they would need all of the time available before the next influenza season to prepare to cope with it adequately.

The conference paid special attention to the question of publicity concerning the Fort Dix findings. On the one hand, they were faced with what was beginning to look like a very serious situation, with important implications for the public; sooner or later public health officials around the country and the world, and the general public itself, would have to be informed. On the other hand, however, no one wished to incite a panic response in the public, especially when the information was still incomplete and so many points needed reconfirmation. The final decision was, therefore, to sit tight and make no announcement for the time being, but wait for the critical confirmation that this really was swine flu at Fort Dix and not a laboratory contaminant: this result was expected within three days. If the laboratory did confirm that it was swine flu virus, then CDC would report the finding factually in its regular *Weekly Morbidity and Mortality Report,* which was due to be released to the press on February 19 and sent out on February 20. At the same time, CDC would inform the appropriate authorities at the World Health Organization and the state and local public health officials with whom it normally maintained very close contact. Finally, the manner in which CDC would make the announcement to the public was discussed, and it was agreed that a statement would be prepared and cleared with the participants later that week.[19]

The report that came from the virology laboratories on February 17 appeared to confirm everyone's worst fears. The virus isolated from the Fort Dix cases was indeed a strain of swine influenza, and the possibility of a chance laboratory contamination had been almost completely ruled out. With this finding, activity moved into a higher gear. BoB, CDC, and NIAID decided to hold another, more expanded emergency meeting at the Bureau of Biologics headquarters in Bethesda, Maryland, just outside of Washington, D.C. This time, in addition to government officials, a number of the country's virological "greats" would be invited, including Kilbourne, Albert Sabin from South Carolina, and members of the Scientific Advisory Committees of CDC and BoB. In addition, representatives of the pharmaceutical manufacturers would be on hand, so that all of the data then available could be reviewed and a tentative course of action planned.

The touchiest issue that week was how to make the announcement to the public. It was agreed that a press conference should be called by CDC in Atlanta and that a low-key announcement should be made, providing only the facts and attempting to avoid a picture of gloom and doom. While attendance at the press conference itself was limited mostly to local reporters, national coverage was assured by setting up a telephone hookup from Atlanta to Washington, where a number of medical reporters and television newsmen were invited to attend. The CDC announcement itself was careful not to mention the 1918 killer flu, but this comparison was brought out during the subsequent question-and-answer period. Nor was this surprising: without the reference to 1918, or to the possibility of pandemic influenza, it would hardly have been a news item worthy of public attention or mention by the national media.

The cat was now out of the bag, however, and that night the three major television networks included brief announcements about swine flu, with the 1918 reference, and one network even showed still pictures of people wearing protective masks during the 1918 epidemic. The next morning, the *New York Times* published a story on its front page by medical reporter Harold Schmeck, headed "U.S. calls flu alert on possible return of epidemic virus" and continuing, "The possibility was raised today that the virus that caused the greatest world epidemic of influenza in modern history . . . the pandemic of 1918–19 may have returned." This type of publicity pained many of the scientists and public health people at CDC and elsewhere, since they felt that there was too much tendency at that time to dwell upon the horrors of the 1918 pandemic. It is difficult, however, to see how it could have been handled otherwise, given the obligation of public officials to provide timely notice of findings of such obvious potential importance, and the obligation of the news media to report these in terms that would be significant to the public. The media did not, after all, invent the 1918 influenza pandemic.

When the February 20 meeting in Bethesda was called to order, little new information was available. All that was known with certainty was that swine flu had hit Fort Dix, causing a number of cases of clinical influenza with one death, and that the ever-widening search for a further outbreak of the disease had thus far yielded no positive results. Yet, a perceptible escalation had taken place in the fears and concerns of the scientists and public health officials in attendance. For reasons that are not entirely clear, the mood seemed to have changed from "What if . . . ?" to "Well, here it is!" There appeared to be almost uniform agreement among both civilian and government scientists that the New Jersey outbreak *might* be the harbinger of more serious and widespread disease to come: while it was impossible to define precisely the extent of the risk involved, everything that they knew about influenza told them that *some* risk of disease spread existed and that it was better to be safe than sorry. The conferees therefore spent much time discussing the logistics of influenza vaccine production and distribution; how much time it would take to field-test and license a vaccine; how fast the manufacturers could mobilize their production facilities and how many doses per egg might be expected; and how a nationwide immunization campaign might be mounted.[20] It was becoming increasingly clear to everyone that if something was going to be done to prepare the country for a possible epidemic that autumn, preparations would have to start fairly soon.

During normal times, the customary procedure for establishing routine immunizations for the civilian population involves recommendations by CDC's Advisory Committee on Immunization Practices (ACIP), a group of outside experts in immunology and infectious diseases appointed by the surgeon general. One of the principal duties of the ACIP is to advise on the strength and composition of vaccines and on who should receive them; CDC then implements these recommendations through its programs with the states. For influenza, the ACIP normally makes its recommendations in January for the flu season starting the next autumn and then meets again in March to review these recommendations. This January, the recommendation had been for a vaccine against A/Victoria (the current flu strain) aimed at the 40 million or so individuals classed as high risks — those over age 65 or with certain chronic diseases. Indeed, the manufactuers had already produced the normal 20 million doses in bulk form and were closing down their production lines.

In view of the Fort Dix outbreak of swine influenza, the March meeting of the ACIP assumed special significance. It was clear that this would be the most important forum for discussing how to respond to the swine flu challenge.

A number of interesting developments had occurred in the two and one-half weeks since the Bethesda meeting. The army had conducted an intensive survey at Fort Dix, and while they did not find any additional active cases of swine influenza, studies of blood samples taken from other recruits showed that as many as five hundred had probably been infected by the swine flu virus, since they showed a positive antibody response to this particular strain. However, the survey by CDC and the New Jersey health officials failed to show any spread of the virus in the surrounding civilian population. Moreover, the nationwide search by state epidemiologists for other cases of swine flu had only turned up a few isolated cases of swine influenza in which human-to-human transmission was considered unlikely, so it was concluded that these infections had resulted from contact with pigs. Outside of the United States, the World Health Organization also reported no outbreaks of swine influenza. Meanwhile, the commercial vaccine manufacturers had tested samples of the Fort Dix virus and found that this strain grew poorly in chick embryos. They would therefore have to await receipt of faster-growing strains, either from Kilbourne in New York or from the CDC laboratories in Atlanta.

All of this information was considered on March 9, when Sencer met with the key members of his staff for an informal discussion of various options, in preparation for the next day's ACIP meeting. It was clear to everyone involved that, while the further spread of swine flu was by no means certain, recommendations for some type of action were in the wind, and it only remained to decide what specifically would be recommended. For the first time, a serious discussion was held about the possibility of recommending large-scale production of swine influenza vaccine, and then stockpiling it until such time as a swine flu outbreak might occur. This option was debated back and forth, but the overriding opinion was that even if all of the vaccine required could be produced by the beginning of the next flu season (September-October), it would probably take eight to ten weeks or longer to distribute and administer the vaccine to a target population many times larger than had ever been attempted before in the history of immunization. In addition, once the vaccine had been delivered into the arms of recipients, it would take at least two weeks for them to develop protective immunity. The program would likely require more than three months to take effect, once the signal to immunize the population had been received. Given the "jet-spread" rapidity of movement that influenza had shown itself capable of in previous epidemics, the consensus was that stockpiling was not a viable option — too many people might sicken and perhaps die while the vaccine was finding its way through the delivery pipeline. As one scientist put it at the time, "Better to store the vaccine in people than in warehouses." Immunization requires two weeks to protect, whereas infection produces disease in only two days.

Sencer's staff also told him that a large-scale campaign to immunize the public might carry with it serious consequences for CDC. It was likely that involvement in such a program would seriously interfere with work on other diseases, disrupting not only CDC itself, but also its other ongoing programs with state health offices. In addition, the institution's image might be threatened. If the pandemic came and, as was quite likely, the program was behind schedule, then millions of people might be screaming for vaccine and blame CDC for the foul-up. On the other hand, if the pandemic did not appear, they would be accused by the public of wasting government money, and it might also cost them the loss of the hard-earned goodwill and respect they had built up among their colleagues in state and local health departments. Potential institutional problems, however, could not be decisive in an organization like CDC. All of the staff there were professionals, deeply committed to the concept of preventive medicine, and swine flu presented a challenge that, at least theoretically, they had the competence, tools, and obligation to meet head-on. This was the message that Sencer received from his staff, and it fell on sympathetic ears.

The March 10 meeting of the Advisory Committee on Immunization Practices was accompanied by an unaccustomed air of barely suppressed excitement and significance. The press was there, and the spotlight was turned on the meeting. In attendance were many of the nation's leading experts on preventive medicine, including Kilbourne who, while not yet a member of the ACIP, was scheduled to join it that summer and would play a significant role in the actions taken that day. The meeting opened with presentations by the technical experts, who summarized the medical, virological, and epidemiological information available up to that point. Several hours of sometimes intense discussion followed, until a consensus emerged on the following points.

1. The Fort Dix outbreak of swine flu was a real one, and a pandemic was possible. While it was somewhat troubling that no further cases had been reported, everyone understood that flu is a curious disease and that the swine flu might be smoldering somewhere in subclinical form, gathering strength and virulence, ready to break out any time. Moreover, Kilbourne's theory of an eleven-year cycle of major pandemics was taken seriously, so the time was approaching for the next round. The big problem was how to estimate the *probability* of a pandemic. No one in the room considered that the chances were negligible, since all were aware that never in the modern history of influenza had a markedly new strain of the virus appeared that was *not* accompanied by pandemic spread. To assign a precise number to this probability was impossible, however, since an estimate had to be based more upon personal judgment than upon scientific fact. The predictions varied considerably, with Kilbourne suggesting that a pandemic was "likely," and other participants guessing (mostly to themselves) figures ranging from about 2 to 20 percent chance of an epidemic.[21]

2. There was no way to estimate the severity of a pandemic, should it appear. The 1918–19 pandemic of Spanish influenza had killed something under 1 percent of those infected, while the death rate in more recent pandemics had been appreciably lower. At Fort Dix, however, there had been one death in twelve cases of swine flu. Although these numbers were too small to be dependable, and few thought that a repetition of the 1918 death rate was likely (especially since antibiotics were now available to

hold down the complications of bacterial pneumonia), no one was willing to go out on a limb to argue that a new pandemic would be a mild one.

3. The normal rules about which segments of the population were at greatest risk might not apply in 1976. The most recent pandemics had shown that the death rate was usually highest in the elderly; since the new virus was swine flu, which had been prevalent in the population for some years after the 1918 pandemic, people over about 50 years of age would be expected to have residual immunity to this strain, whereas those under 50 would be unprotected. In addition, the new virus was a swine flu strain, which had imposed an unusually high mortality on young adults during the 1918 pandemic. Since the greater susceptibility of the elderly might be balanced by their residual immunity, whereas the younger population would have no protection at all, the entire population might be at equal risk during the next pandemic, and therefore everyone would require protective immunization.

4. This was the first time since 1957 that the early warning signal of an impending pandemic had been received in time to do something about it. In 1976, with the experience gained from earlier years, vaccines were safer and more effective, and modern "jet guns" could deliver the vaccine far more rapidly and painlessly than was previously possible using syringes and needles. If a decision were made right away, the manufacturers would have time to order eggs and go into large-scale production, so that inoculations might begin prior to the onset of the autumn flu season. Not only would each additional person immunized be protected, thus reducing morbidity and mortality, but that immune person would also be removed from the chain of viral contagion, thus indirectly protecting others. If enough individuals could be immunized, the development of a "herd immunity" might possibly interrupt the spread of the virus and protect the entire population. For influenza, the protective effect of herd immunity was estimated to operate when some 60 to 70 percent of the entire population was immune to it.

It was clear, then, that large-scale immunization would be recommended by the ACIP, even though nothing on this scale and with this timing had ever been attempted before in the history of preventive medicine. Once again, this required discussion of the probable efficacy and safety of a new vaccine. Since the swine flu strain of virus should be no different in principle from any of the other new vaccine strains used previously, the experts predicted that the new vaccine would probably show the typical 50 to 80 percent protection rate experienced in prior years. A broad review of the medical literature on flu vaccine side-effects by CDC epidemiologist Michael Hattwicke suggested that there was little to worry about on this score. While many sore arms and fevers could be anticipated, and some coincidental heart attacks and other mishaps might occur, few serious complications were likely, and these were part of the accepted price of any large-scale immunization campaign.[22]

The decision by the ACIP to recommend positive action on swine flu was unanimous. Only one member, Dr. Russell Alexander, of the University of Washington School of Public Health, raised the question about the possibility of stockpiling the vaccine until a clearer signal emerged for its inoculation into people. He felt that one should always be conservative about putting foreign material into the human body, especially when the number of bodies approached 200 million. Furthermore, he pointed out that once the pandemic started, it would be much easier to mobilize the public, since everyone would move faster when faced by the real thing. He also wanted to know, "At what point do we stop going on with our preparations to immunize everybody and turn to stockpiling instead — what point in terms both of progress of our preparations and progress of the disease?" New Jersey's Goldfield, although he was not a member of the committee, approved of Alexander's points, and later "went public" in opposition to the swine flu immunization program.

Since he was normally a mild-mannered individual, Alexander did not make a passionate speech in favor of these points; instead, he voiced his opinions through questions or comments when the opportunity presented, so they made little impression on the group. The arguments about the rapid spread of influenza pandemics and the difficulty of cranking up the public health machinery to immunize substantially the entire U.S. population appeared so convincing to the others that this point was not explored further. During one of the breaks in the meeting, the three top government officials present, Sencer, Meyer, and Seal, discussed the stockpile option, apart from the others. Someone made the point, understandable to any upper-level career civil servant, "Suppose there is a pandemic accompanied by deaths. Then it comes out that they had the opportunity to save life; they made the vaccine, and then put it into the refrigerator! That translates to 'they did nothing' and worse, they didn't even recommend an immunization campaign to the Secretary [of Health, Education and Welfare]."[23]

The minutes of the ACIP meeting record the following conclusion: "It was, therefore, agreed that the production of vaccine must proceed and that a plan for vaccine administration be developed."[24]

It is difficult to evaluate all of the complex factors that enter into a decision of this type. Those who participated in the meetings on swine flu during the course of the decision-making process insist that the principal factor guiding the actions of everyone involved was a real concern for the public welfare — and there seems to be little reason to doubt this. It is, after all, the formal duty of those in government, from CDC and BoB up to the president, to protect the health of the American people. For their part, the civilian scientists, so long supported by public funds, felt a deep obligation to justify that support, and to show that their science was indeed useful to humanity. As one man later recalled, this seemed a good opportunity to repay society for all it had done for him as a public health doctor.

But other, more personal factors must have contributed to the decision, and these are also worth our attention. A public official might not only feel an obligation to protect the health of the people but might also suspect that a wrong decision on such an important issue might cost him his job. If he failed to act, and an influenza pandemic did appear, might he not be indicted for negligence or stupidity? Far better to act positively, and run the lesser risk that if a pandemic failed to come, he could only be accused of wasting the taxpayers' money (almost a forgivable sin in government). On another level, the CDC was located far from the center of power in Washington, and it had seen its preventive medicine budget whittled down year after year under the parsimonious Nixon and Ford administrations. Its director might view involvement in a swine flu immunization campaign as a chance to show how effective his agency could be and just how important its preventive medicine mission was in the national health picture. Or consider the influenza virologist, normally confined to his narrow circle of fellow specialists, who must now have felt a secret thrill of anticipation at seeing his subject in the forefront and in newspaper headlines, and at finally being able to show the general public how important his science really was in the grand scheme of things. Similarly, the specialist in preventive medicine and public health would have been less than human not to feel a certain elation at the prospect of showing, in so significant a fashion, what disease control and epidemiology were capable of doing for the health of the people.

In a general sense, these factors are part of the politics of people and of science, and they played the same significant yet immeasurable role in decision-making at this level that more classical politics would play when the swine flu question was considered in Washington.

CHAPTER 4

Making Public Policy:
Political Implementation

D AVID Sencer was known as a tough, competent bureaucrat. He ran a very tight ship at the Center for Disease Control, and little of importance happened there that he did not know about and influence. He had large ambitions for himself, large ambitions for his agency, and a deep commitment to its mission — preventive medicine. Within CDC, his staff often complained that he held the reins too tightly and pushed them too hard, but most were devoted to him; outside of CDC, he was sometimes suspected of being wily, and too much of an "operator."

The challenge posed by the swine flu outbreak was one that a self-confident activist like Sencer would have relished, for both institutional and personal reasons. Not only did his position require him to act to protect the health of the American people, but here was also an almost unique opportunity to show the world just how efficient he and his agency could be. The scientists on the Advisory Committee on Immunization Practices had recommended large-scale production of vaccine and the development of a plan for administration of the vaccine, with the clear implication of major government involvement: now it was up to CDC to implement these recommendations.

Sencer had worked in government for a long time, and he knew how difficult it was, within the federal bureaucracy, to obtain a clear and *rapid* decision to act. He saw that the problem was made doubly difficult by the need for new moneys to support an immunization program, since the Ford administration had imposed tight budgetary constraints during the recent past, and any new funds would require legislative action in the Congress. The problem was further complicated because decision making would quickly pass beyond those levels of bureaucracy peopled by health professionals and would increasingly involve bureaucrats whose main concern had less to do with health and science than with budgets and their political implications. But Sencer knew how the system worked and how to frame an urgent request for action which might work its way successfully up through a bureaucracy at each of whose levels it was easier (and

34

often safer) to object to a new program than to support it. Since he agreed so strongly with his scientific advisers on the magnitude of the threat of a swine flu pandemic, and since he felt that firm and rapid government involvement was the only way to meet this threat effectively, Sencer set about preparing a document that would command attention and ensure agreement. The issues could be posed and the solutions offered in such a way as to counter the objections that he knew might be raised, and to render the final actions politically irresistible.

Sencer finished his swine flu memorandum on March 13, and immediately called his superior, Assistant Secretary of HEW for Health, Dr. Theodore Cooper, to advise him of the ACIP recommendation and to let him know that a recommendation for a national swine flu immunization program was on its way to Washington. In addition, Sencer notified John Seal and Harry Meyer about the contents and implications of the memorandum, and asked them to double-check with their scientific advisers, as he would with the ACIP members, to be sure that the scientific community was behind this recommendation for federal action.

The Action Memorandum

In typical bureaucratic fashion, the recommendations that Sencer prepared took the form of a memorandum to the secretary of Health, Education, and Welfare, Dr. David Mathews, from the assistant secretary for health. While Sencer might be the boss at CDC in Atlanta with his own large staff, within the HEW bureaucracy he was only one of six agency heads responsible to Assistant Secretary Cooper, and thus, in a sense, was Cooper's No. 1 staff man for disease control and preventive medicine. The director of CDC is considered by the hierarchy to be a career "technician," whereas the Assistant Secretary, while a health professional, represents the lowest level of political appointment and is, therefore, the appropriate person to recommend and to take responsibility for official government policy.

The title of Sencer's action memorandum was "Swine Influenza — Action." It started out by presenting the "Issue: How should the federal government respond to the influenza problem caused by a new virus?" We will touch here only on the salient points of this memorandum, but it does deserve to be read in its entirety, and it is included in full as Appendix A. It is an interesting document, first because it provides an excellent example of effective bureaucratic writing, and second, because it survived unchanged as *the* definitive recommendation throughout the bureaucratic chain of command and into the office of the president.

The Sencer memorandum began with a statement of the facts:

1. In February 1976, a new strain of influenza virus . . . was isolated from an outbreak of disease among recruits in training at Fort Dix, New Jersey.
2. The virus is antigenically related to the influenza virus which has been implicated as the cause of the 1918–1919 pandemic which killed 450,000 people — more than 400 of every 100,000 Americans.
3. The entire U.S. population under the age of 50 is probably susceptible to this new strain.
4. . . . . Since 1930, the virus has been limited to transmission among swine . . . with no secondary person-to-person transmission.
5. In an average year, influenza causes about 17,000 deaths (9 per 100,000 population) and costs the nation approximately $500 million.
6. Severe epidemics, or pandemics, of influenza occur at approximately ten-year intervals. In 1968–69, influenza struck 20 percent of our population, causing more than 33,000 deaths (14 per 100,000) and cost an estimated $3.2 billion.
7. A vaccine to protect against swine influenza can be developed before the next flu season. . . .

All of the important facts are here, and are presented in a form that the layman can understand. Of equal importance, they contain many points that would appeal to the politician: the implied new threat to the health of the American people; the cost in disease and death that influenza had brought in the past; and the impressive financial cost to the country as a whole that accompanies both normal and abnormal outbreaks of influenza disease. Here at the very beginning of the memorandum is all the excuse that any bureaucrat or politician would want to approve an immunization program: the protection of the health of the American people and the saving of their money. While CDC and civilian scientists were later to object to what they called the overemphasis by Secretary Mathews, President Ford, and the news media of the horrors of the 1918 pandemic, this connection surfaced whenever swine flu was discussed in 1976, and was even made explicit in Sencer's second "fact." Indeed, without reference to 1918, neither the ACIP recommendations nor the actions that followed it would have been comprehensible.

The memorandum next took up a set of "Assumptions":

1. Although there has been only one outbreak of A/swine influenza, person-to-person spread has been proven and additional outbreaks cannot be ruled out. Present evidence and past experience indicate a strong possibility that this country will experience widespread A/swine influenza in 1976–1977. Swine flu represents a major antigenic shift from recent viruses. . . . These are the ingredients for pandemic.

2. Routine public health influenza recommendations (immunization of the population at high risk) would not forestall a flu pandemic. Routine actions would have to be supplemented.
3. The situation is one of "go or no-go." If extraordinary measures are to be undertaken, there is barely enough time to assure adequate vaccine production and to mobilize the nation's health-care delivery system. . . . A decision must be made now.
4. There is no medical epidemiologic basis for excluding any part of the population — swine flu vaccine will be recommended for the total population. . . . Further, it is assumed that it would be socially and politically unacceptable to *plan* for less than 100 percent coverage. Therefore, it is assumed that any recommendation for action must be directed toward the goal of immunizing 213 million people in three months. . . . The nation has never attempted an immunization program of such scope and intensity.
5. A public health undertaking of this magnitude cannot succeed without Federal leadership, sponsorship, and some level of financial support.
6. . . . Nationally, the vaccine will cost in excess of $100 million. To this total must be added delivery costs, as well as costs relating to surveillance and monitoring. . . . It will be extremely difficult to estimate the amount of additional costs that will result from a crash influenza immunization program.
7. The Advisory Committee on Immunization Practices will recommend, formally and publicly, the immunization of the total U.S. population against A/swine influenza.
8. Any recommended course of action, other than no action, must assure:
   — that a supply of vaccine is produced which is adequate to immunize the whole population;
   — that adequate supplies of vaccine are available as needed to health-care delivery points;
   — that the American people are made aware of the need for immunization . . .;
   — . . . that the Public Health Service maintain . . . surveillance of the population for complications of vaccination . . .;
   — that the unique research opportunities be maximized;
   — that evaluation of the effectiveness of the efforts is conducted.

It is clear from the way in which these assumptions are presented that the writer is biased in favor of action and is seeking to justify this action. All of his instincts, and all of the advice of his scientific advisers and staff, told Sencer that this was the correct line to take. In addition, hidden away in the last few items in assumption 8 was the reflection of a different special interest, which went beyond the immediate problem of protecting the public from a flu pandemic. An effective national immunization campaign would not only justify and strengthen preventive medicine but would also provide unique scientific opportunities in other areas — opportunities which were almost irresistible to the professionals and which had been discussed in the different scientific meetings. Thus, the epidemiologist would have a distinctive opportunity to demonstrate the value of his profession and also to refine and extend the tools of his trade. The virologist could see additional financial support in the program, and unique research opportunities that would permit him to improve his knowledge of the nature and action of the influenza virus. Finally, the public health professional could view the program not only in terms of its immediate benefits in preventing influenza but also as a novel social experiment in preventive medicine on a scale never before possible.

The next section of the action memorandum then discussed alternative courses of action. This included a set of four options couched in terms that are not unusual either inside or outside of government: while all are presented with the appearance of impartiality, the option favored by the writer is designed to be accepted, and the alternatives are subtly designed to be rejected. The first option was "no action," and was accompanied by a set of "pros" and "cons." Among the pros were: "The marketplace would prevail. . . . The pandemic might not occur, and the Department would have avoided unnecessary health expenditures. . . . Any real action would require direct federal intervention which is contrary to current administration philosophy." Among the cons were "Congress, the media, and the American people will expect some action. . . . The Administration can tolerate unnecessary health expenditures better than unnecessary death and illness. . . . In all likelihood, Congress will act on its own initiative." The arguments against "no action" were convincing to the politician, especially the points that "the American people will expect" and "Congress will act." In 1976 and earlier, the Democratic Congress had often been at loggerheads with the Republican White House, repeatedly accusing President Ford of indecisiveness and lack of leadership, especially in domestic social areas. No administration would be happy at seeing the opposition party in Congress taking credit for defending the health of the American people, if the pandemic should arrive as predicted.

The second alternative was a "minimum response." Under this option, there would be a limited federal role, with the government restricted to advising manufacturers, stimulating local health organizations, and helping to educate the public. Among the points in favor of this course of action were "high visibility, [but] minimum federal intervention. . . . The burden on the federal budget would be minimal. . . . Success would depend upon widespread voluntary action. . . ." But the arguments against the minimal response option appeared convincing. "There is little assurance that vaccine manufacturers will undertake the massive production effort. . . . There would be no control over the distribution of vaccines. . . . The poor . . . and the aging usually get left out. . . . Probably only about half the population would get immunized." This was the course followed in 1957, with very unhappy results.

The third option presented was based upon total government responsibility for a national immunization program. The government would take over the purchase and distribution of vaccines to state health departments, and vaccines would only be available through highly publicized governmental programs. In this option's favor it was pointed out that this would be the best way to assure widespread availability of vaccine and equitable distribution throughout the nation, with access to immunization services not dependent upon economic status. Arguments against this option included its greater cost (some $190 million) and the inefficiency that would result from the failure to take advantage of the health delivery system of the private sector. In addition, the telling point was made that a totally public (i.e., government-run) program would be contrary to the spirit and customs of health-care delivery in this country. This last item would be taken seriously by a Republican administration.

The fourth option presented was termed a "combined approach." Logically, it should really have come third in the hierarchy of federal options, between "minimal response" and "total government responsibility." But no good memorandum writer would bury his favored solution in the middle — far better to raise and shoot down the straw men first, and then come to the rescue with an attractive last option.

The preferred solution would "take advantage of the strengths and resources of both the public and private sectors." It was based upon federal purchase of vaccine for all citizens, safety and efficacy testing by the BoB, field trials and research by NIAID, and distribution and final immunization of the public by a mix of state, local, and private medical services. The arguments in favor of this option were presented convincingly. These not only included efficiency of distribution and administration and the availability of vaccine to all citizens independent of socioeconomic factors but also mentioned the politically understandable point that "undertaking the program in this manner provides a practical, contemporary example of government, industry, and private citizens cooperating to serve a common cause." The estimated cost of this program, requiring a supplemental request to Congress, was approximately $134 million, of which $100 million was estimated for vaccine at fifty cents per dose, $26 million for distribution and publicity, and $8 million for surveillance and research.

In the discussion of the program, Sencer pointed out that "we have not undertaken a health program of this scope and intensity before in our history. There are no precedents, nor mechanisms in place that are suited to an endeavor of this magnitude." In strongly recommending the fourth option, it was argued that "the magnitude of the challenge suggests that the Department must either be willing to take extraordinary steps or be willing to accept an approach to the problem that cannot succeed."

Assent in HEW

Time was of the essence. If Sencer hoped to get action on a swine flu immunization program and meet the deadlines imposed by vaccine production, testing, and distribution timetables before the onset of the flu season in September, then he would have to move the memorandum personally through the HEW hierarchy. He completed the document on Saturday, March 13, and appeared with it in Washington the following Monday morning. His immediate superior, Assistant Secretary for Health Cooper, was in Egypt that day, keeping a long-standing engagement, but he knew and approved of Sencer's recommendation, which they had discussed over the phone. Prior to his departure, Cooper had arranged with his deputy assistant secretary, Dr. James Dickson, to take charge of the influenza problem in his absence. Cooper had even arranged to be contacted in Egypt through the extensive world-wide communication facilities of the White House, if his help was needed.

The first step in the procedure occurred at the regular daily staff meeting in the office of HEW Secretary David Mathews. As was the custom, they would go around the table, with each official briefing the secretary on new developments and problems in his office. When Dickson's turn came, he outlined the events that had occurred at Fort Dix, the discussions that had taken place at CDC, and their implications for the department and for the country, following fairly closely the points made in Sencer's action memorandum. Everyone around the table realized immediately what all of this implied, and while "We all understood the pandemic might not come," serious discussion was preempted by anecdotes of what had happened in 1918.

Immediately after the staff meeting, Mathews asked to see Sencer in order to get more information. Expecting this, Dickson had alerted Harry Meyer of BoB, and the four of them met to discuss the issue further. Sencer argued his case forcefully, even going beyond the substance of the action memorandum, since he felt that Mathews might be the most difficult person to convince in the entire chain of the federal hierarchy. Mathews had been Secretary of HEW for only seven months, having been summoned to Washington by President Ford from the presidency of the University of Alabama. His comparative youth, combined with a soft

Southern drawl and the graceful demeanor of a southern gentleman of the old school, caused many in Washington to suspect him of being ineffectual — a "political lightweight." Above all, the Public Health Service people in his own department suspected that he was uninformed and uninterested in their affairs and that he lacked influence in the higher circles of the administration to get things done on their behalf. In addition, federal health programs in general, and Sencer's CDC in particular, had suffered over the years at the hands of first Nixon's and then Ford's budget slashers, both within HEW and in the White House Office of Management and Budget. Sencer thus went in fearing that the immunization program was threatened more by its cost than by charges of "excessive governmental interference."

The Health Service people underestimated Secretary Mathews. He did, in fact, know something about influenza, and was favorably inclined toward preventive medicine to the extent that he understood it, and especially toward preventive immunization, a theory he felt he understood well. As soon as Dickson finished summarizing the issue, Mathews asked what the probability of pandemic was. When Dickson said "Unknown," he knew "from the look on Mathews' face when I said that, you could take it for granted that this decision was going to be made." Mathews questioned Sencer and Meyer closely on two issues: the probability of a pandemic and the possibility that enough safe vaccine could be manufactured and administered. Neither could put a number on the probability, but both agreed it was greater than zero. On the second question, both agreed that it would be "a hell of a job," but it could be done if the decision were made soon enough. During the course of those discussions, Meyer felt somewhat uncomfortable at Sencer's "hard sell" approach to Secretary Mathews; he felt that the information they had should speak for itself. Meyer, concerned with the public response if a pandemic should fail to appear, stressed the importance of bringing as many people as possible into a consensus for decision-making, a practice that he followed assiduously within his own agency. We see here an interesting contrast in the personalities of these two government scientists: Sencer is by nature self-confident, brash, and ready to push a program or a decision to its utmost, while Meyer is more cautious and quiet, always seeking broad outside consensus to support his actions, and continuously reexamining their validity.[25]

In the final analysis, Mathews was not hard to convince of the need for a national immunization program. As we have seen, Mathews favored the substance of the program on its own merits, but his second reason for endorsing the program is even more interesting. Mathews recalls: "As soon as I heard about swine flu and its implications for a pandemic, I realized that the political system would have to respond. There was no way out, as long as all of the scientists supported it. We had to assume a probability greater than zero, and that's all that we needed to know. You can't face the electorate later, if the pandemic arrives, and say that the probability was so low that the costs outweighed the benefits. The people would never forgive us."

The appointment of a member of the president's cabinet is a political one. The secretary has large numbers of specialists and technicians who know about programmatic details and how the department functions technically — the secretary's job is concerned with the broader political picture: interrelationships with other departments, relationships with Congress, the philosophical approach of the president, the public perception of government programs, and finally and not least important, the reelection needs of the president and the party. Whatever else Mathews's shortcomings in running so cumbersome an agency as HEW, his words show that during his seven months in Washington he had at least learned this most fundamental of its political guidelines.

That same morning, Mathews wrote a note to James Lynn, director of the Office of Management and Budget (OMB), to advise him that a request for new funds was on its way. In recent years, the OMB had become an all-important arm of the presidency, since it was not only responsible for devising and overseeing the budget of the United States government, but lately it had begun more and more to evaluate programs within the government departments, wielding a fiscal stick to insure that the president's wishes and political philosophy were translated correctly. The ground rules required OMB's approval for an undertaking of this type.

Secretary Mathews's note to OMB Director Lynn is interesting:

> There is evidence there will be a major flu epidemic this coming fall. The indication is that we will see a return of the 1918 flu virus that is the most virulent form of flu. In 1918, a half-million people died. The projections are that this virus will kill one million Americans in 1976.
>
> To have adequate protection, industry would have to be advised now in order to have time to prepare the some 200 million doses of vaccine required for mass inoculation. The decision will have to be made in the next week or so. We will have a recommendation on this matter since a supplemental appropriation will be required. . . .

This note was written on March 15, only five days after the ACIP meeting, but the change in tone was marked, and the stakes had gone up substantially. Five days earlier in Atlanta, most of the scientists spoke of some possibility of a pandemic. Sencer's action memorandum three days later used the term *strong possibility*. Now Mathews had changed the "possible" into a "will be." In speaking of the present virus, the scientists and Sencer described it as antigenically related to the 1918 virus; in turn, Mathews translated this to OMB as "a return of the 1918 flu virus." Finally, although the scientists repeatedly said that they had no way of assessing the virulence or severity of the new virus, Mathews extrapolated the half-million deaths in 1918 to a projection of one million deaths in 1976, since the population had almost doubled. This is an interesting escalation of fears about the new virus in so short a time. It undoubtedly reflected the growing sense of uncertainty and urgency which infected all concerned and which increased with each retelling of the story. It may also reflect, in part, one of the important realities of any large organization, espcially true of government: the higher up one goes in a hierarchy, the more the specialist gives way to the generalist, and the more the specific facts give way to nonspecific generalities and impressions. Government officials usually know that the higher the level at which a decision is sought, the simpler and starker and more compelling must be the presentation — a factor that may have affected the terms in which Sencer's memorandum and Mathews's note were couched.

The Mathews note did not take OMB by surprise. Victor Zafra, the chief of OMB's health examiners, had read the original report of swine flu in the *New York Times* of February 20, and realized that it was only a matter of time before some request for money would surface from CDC. While OMB was normally suspicious of Sencer and of many CDC programs, they were, necessarily, political realists. They knew that any program (and especially one receiving widespread public attention) that posed an urgent choice between spending money or putting lives at risk could have only one answer — spend the money. This was reflected in an internal OMB memorandum that did not even raise the question of not approving the program, but rather restricted itself to the possibility of reprogramming existing Public Health Service funds and to questioning the validity of the final figure of $134 million.

It was clear that the die had been cast. A decision to go ahead with a national immunization campaign was inevitable. The nature of the swine flu threat, its inherent unpredictability, and especially the wording of Sencer's action memorandum forced the hand of everyone involved. At the lower levels of the bureaucracy, an understanding of the scientific realities indicated that it could and *should* be done; at the higher levels, an understanding of the political realities indicated that it *must* be done.

CHAPTER 5

Making Public Policy: Presidential Decision

S PRING is an interesting season in Washington every year, but during election years it is doubly interesting. Those officials who were successful in following Everett Dirksen's famous First Law of Politics — get elected — are now busy in pursuit of his Second Law — get reelected. Suddenly, newspapers and television reports are filled with items showing how government is responding to the will of the people: taxes are cut; pork barrel measures pass the Congress that include public works projects in key states and congressional districts; programs are announced to make government more efficient and to "reduce the fat" in the military or in the bureaucracy. But above all, those up for reelection issue proclamations and take actions designed to show them as the statesmen they really are and to correct any erroneous impression to the contrary which the electorate might have received since the previous election.

In all of these respects, 1976 was a typical election year in Washington. In addition to the election of the full House of Representatives and some one-third of the Senators, however, it was a presidential election year in which Gerald Ford, who had succeeded the deposed Richard Nixon in 1974, was running for a full term in his own right. The presidential primaries were now under way, and Ford was being troubled by the strong candidacy of Ronald Reagan for the Republican nomination. In the first primary in New Hampshire in February, Ford had only narrowly defeated Reagan, but he had picked up strength in the next four primaries, inflicting a telling defeat on Reagan in Florida on March 9. However, the next primary was in North Carolina on March 23, where Reagan was showing uncomfortable strength, and where in fact he would shake up the Ford campaign by winning. Throughout this period, both Reagan and the opposition Democrats continued to harp on one principal theme: the Ford presidency was weak and indecisive. It was in this context that swine flu, far from being Ford's biggest problem in March of 1976, appeared on the president's desk.

The first notice that President Ford received of the HEW request for supplemental funds for the swine flu program occurred on the afternoon of March 15, when he met with OMB's Lynn, his deputy Paul O'Neill, and with James Cavanaugh, deputy director of the Domestic Council, who was responsible for staff assistance to the president in areas such as health. Cavanaugh had already heard about swine flu from Theodore Cooper, who had called to alert him before he left for Egypt. In addition, according to good staff practices, he had been alerted by OMB's O'Neill and had also received the Sencer memorandum from Dickson.

In the manner of a good staff man getting ready for a new issue that "the Boss" must deal with, Cavanaugh had done some preliminary checking on his own. Any senior staff man in Washington will have an informal network of trustworthy consultants to sound out on a given issue, and Cavanaugh's consultant in health was his old boss, Dr. Charles Edwards, who had been Cooper's predecessor as assistant secretary for health in the Nixon administration. Edwards said that from what he had heard of the swine flu affair, Sencer's recommendation seemed to be the only possible course. When Cavanaugh later received the same message from Assistant Secretary Cooper, whom he also trusted, it became clear that the president would receive no negative signals on this issue from within the White House.

Several days later, Secretary Mathews again brought up the swine flu problems with the president, and it was agreed to have a full review of the issue the following week. The meeting took place at the White House on Monday morning, March 22. It would have been one of many in the president's busy day, and was allowed thirty minutes on his schedule. In typical fashion, a briefing paper was prepared for the president by one of the staff (in this case of OMB, since it involved a request for new funds). It contained a thumbnail outline of the issue and a list of "talking points" to provide the president with a point of departure for the discussion. The briefing paper was accompanied by the expected copy of Sencer's action memorandum and an attachment entitled "Uncertainties Surrounding a Federal Mass Swine Flu Immunization Program," which reflected OMB's discomfort. The attachment raised questions about: the real probability of a pandemic occurring; the possibility that another mutation of the flu virus might appear next autumn, against which the new vaccine might not be effective; the seriousness of the epidemic if it did come; whether such a mass immunization program in 1976 might not imply similar programs in other years; and whether the scientific community fully agreed with the Sencer recommendation.

The president's meeting was attended by Secretary Mathews, Assistant Secretary Cooper (who had just the day before returned from abroad), OMB's Lynn and O'Neill, the Domestic Council's director, James Cannon, together with Cavanaugh and his health assistant, Spencer Johnson, and White House Chief of Staff, Richard Cheney. The president appeared quite interested in the entire issue, and asked probing questions: What was the exact probability of a serious epidemic developing? How many people were likely to get sick, and how serious would the disease be? Would they really be able to produce and distribute enough vaccine by the start of the next flu season?

The experts were forced to confess that they did not really know what the probability was of a pandemic appearing that autumn, and if it did appear, what its severity might be. But they did convince the president that the threat was real, and that for almost the first time, public health officials were in a position to head off an epidemic on a national scale. The president was assured that enough vaccine could be made in time and that enough fertilized eggs would be available to grow the large amount of virus vaccine needed — on this point even the secretary of agriculture had been reassuring, stating that "the roosters of America are ready to do their duty."

As happened at so many other discussions of this question, much attention was paid to the political implications of a decision to act or not to act. If the pandemic did not come, President Ford would be accused of having wasted the taxpayers' money and of having spread false alarms — in brief, of having made yet another erroneous judgment. If they acted and the pandemic did come, any inadequacy or mix-up in the production and distribution of vaccine would be laid at the president's door — another example of ineffectual leadership. But the overwhelming consideration was that if they failed to act and a pandemic came, then the worst accusation of all might be leveled at the president — that he let people get sick and die because he thought more of balancing the budget than of the welfare of the public. As one participant told the president, it was a no-win situation politically, and no good would come of it as far as the election was concerned. The news media and the public already knew about the Fort Dix outbreak, and about the predictions of the scientists. Many people, both inside and outside of government, knew about the Sencer action memorandum. If they failed to act, the memorandum would surely be leaked to the press very soon, and cause a public uproar that would pose serious problems for the election campaign. In the view of some, the Sencer memorandum was "a gun to our heads." But this analogy seems to be somewhat misplaced — the bad news was the swine flu outbreak itself, and it seems inappropriate to lay the blame for it on the messenger.

Given the circumstances, the decision was inevitable. As the President concluded: "I think you ought to gamble on the side of caution. I would always rather be ahead of the curve than behind it. I had a lot of confidence in Ted Cooper and Dave Mathews. They had kept me informed from the time this was discovered. Now Ted Cooper was advocating an early start in immunization, as fast as we could go, especially in children and old people. So that was what we ought to do, unless there were some major technical objection." [26]

Since the decision was to go ahead, the next question was whether, in view of the political "no-win" uncertainties of the program, someone other than the President ought to make the public announcement. Mathews offered to do so as secretary of HEW, and even Cooper might have made the announcement as the nation's highest-ranking doctor. But the president appeared pleased and even eager to sponsor the swine flu program himself. In part, he felt that it was his duty to lend the weight of his office to a national program of this magnitude. In part, he may also have felt that the decision was politically correct, since it would help counter the accusations of indecisive leadership. The decision to make the swine flu program a presidential one was probably inevitable, although it was to have serious implications in the months to come. When the president announced the target of immunizing the entire population by a given date, he put his prestige on the line and thereby deprived his subordinates of all freedom of action to modify these goals — even as production and insurance problems developed later and as month after month went by with no further cases of swine flu appearing anywhere in the world. Had Mathews or Cooper made the initial announcement of the program, it is likely that the history of the swine flu immunization campaign of 1976 would have taken a far different course.

Curiously, no final decision emerged from the meeting of March 22, although it is clear that President Ford had decided to act. There then occurred one of those interesting set pieces so typical of the Washington scene. There is a reasonable premise that if one is going to do something in any event, then it might just as well be done in a style designed to obtain as much credibility, as well as political mileage, as possible for both the program and the sponsor. In any area, but especially in health and in science, this means appealing to the authority of the acknowledged leaders in the field — those who are known in Washington as the "poobahs." Even though the president had been assured that all of the leading experts in the country were in favor of a swine flu immunization program, he requested a meeting two days later with the nation's top scientists. This meeting would be attended not only by actively involved influenza and public health scientists but also by Doctors Jonas Salk and Albert Sabin of polio vaccine fame. The meeting was designed both to demonstrate to the country that the president's decision was based upon the best scientific advice and also to serve the important purpose of forcing the scientists to commit themselves to the program in public, and, therefore, to share any blame that might accrue if something went wrong later on. In addition, the meeting had another interesting purpose. For almost a quarter of a century, Sabin and Salk had been in continuous and often almost violent scientific opposition to each other, starting with the battle between Salk's killed polio vaccine and Sabin's live attenuated-virus vaccine. It was widely known that these two cordially detested each other, so that if both would come to the White House and openly agree on the advisability of the swine flu immunization campaign, this could be taken as almost a sure sign that it should be undertaken.

The second White House meeting on swine flu took place in the Cabinet Room on March 24 at 3:30 p.m. In prompt response to this impressive invitation, scientists had hastened to Washington from all over the country. In addition, there were representatives from the American Medical Association, state health officials, and large numbers of White House and HEW aides. The president indicated that he had called upon them to solicit their advice, and Sencer then presented a review of the salient facts. Next he consulted Salk, who strongly supported the mass immunization campaign. Salk saw it both as a great opportunity to combat an important disease and at the same time help to educate the public in preventive medicine and also as a means to justify further basic research. Then Sabin spoke in enthusiastic support of the immunization program. The president went around the table, questioning the experts and indicating a serious concern about the subject. While all of the scientists were pleased by Ford's interest and gratified by the opportunity to attend so high level a meeting, many had the feeling that they were being used and that the discussion was pro forma, since the decision seemed already to have been made. Whatever the case, the president finally asked for a show of hands on whether or not to proceed with the immunization campaign, and all hands went up. He urged possible dissenters to voice any objections they might have, but none were forthcoming. Then, in quite an unusual move, the president recessed the meeting, indicating that he would be in his oval office should anyone wish to express any private doubts about the program. No one came. A short time later, the president returned to the Cabinet Room, thanked the participants, and invited Sabin and Salk to accompany him to the Press Room, where he would make his announcement.

President Ford's announcement of the swine flu immunization campaign was well attended by the national press and television. That morning, many of the leading medical reporters who operate out of Washington had received an unusual call from the White House, alerting them that an important announcement of interest to them would be made that afternoon. When they arrived, they found that a swine flu "fact sheet" for the announcement had been distributed *while the president was still consulting in the Cabinet Room.*

With Salk and Sabin on either side of him at the microphone, the president made his announcement:

> I have just concluded a meeting on a subject of vast importance to all Americans. . . . I have been advised that there is a very real possibility that unless we take counteractions, there could be an epidemic of this dangerous disease [swine flu] next fall and winter here in the United States. . . . at this time, no one knows exactly how serious this threat could be. Nevertheless, we cannot afford to take a chance with the health of our nation. Accordingly . . . I am asking the Congress to appropriate $135 million, prior to their April recess, for the production of sufficient vaccine to inoculate every man, woman, and child in the United States.[27]

When questions were invited, the reporters concentrated on two main subjects. Since the president had suffered a stunning defeat the day before to Ronald Reagan in the North Carolina primary, the immediate question was: Was this announcement political? Sabin, Mathews, and Cooper all emphasized that the threat was real and that the president had to act.

The second concern of the reporters was one that had vexed everyone who had heard of swine flu, from Fort Dix to Atlanta to Washington: What was the probability of a pandemic coming, and how serious would it be? Sencer had asked this question of his scientific advisers, Cooper had asked it of Sencer, Mathews had asked it of Cooper, and the president has asked it of everyone. In this modern age of science, when scientists could manipulate the atom, put a man on the moon, or break the genetic code, why were they not able to answer this seemingly simple question? To understand the entire swine flu affair of 1976, it is necessary to appreciate the shortcomings of the science of influenza, and for this we must take a brief look at the molecular biology of this strange virus.

CHAPTER 6

Influenza,
the Impure Science

M ICROBIOLOGISTS have always had great difficulty in knowing how to classify viruses, which exist somewhere in that hazy region between living creatures and inanimate objects. They are, on the one hand, fairly simple structures that can be crystallized from solution like any simple molecule, and they lack the complex biological machinery necessary for reproducing themselves which even the most primitive plants and animals possess. They do, however, have the ability to penetrate the cells of susceptible hosts, where they take over the genetic machinery of the infected cell and force it to synthesize new virus. This is possible because the virus particle contains within its simple gene structure all of the information, but none of the machinery, required to reproduce itself. It succeeds by inserting this information into the elaborate machinery of the infected cell, subverting it into producing foreign virus rather than native substances.

In its outward features, the influenza virus is not much different from other viruses. The electron microscope (figure 6) shows the virus to be roughly spherical in shape, with a large number of small projections sticking out from its surface. A diagrammatic representation of the influenza virus (shown in figure 7) makes its components easier to understand. In the central core of the virus particle are eight genes, composed of ribose nucleic acid (RNA), which carry all of the genetic information of the virus. In addition, the core contains proteins, which differ among the major influenza types, A, B, and C. Around this core is the surface membrane, which holds the virus together, and from whose surface project a large number of protein molecules that look like spikes. The pointed spikes are called hemagglutinin (H), so named because they have specific receptors on them that enable them to bind to red blood cells and to clump or agglutinate them. The blunt-ended spikes, called neuraminidase (N), possess a specialized enzymatic activity.

The hemagglutinin and neuraminidase components of the influenza virus are of extreme importance to our story, since they play key roles in influenza infection. It is the specific receptor on the hemagglutinin that

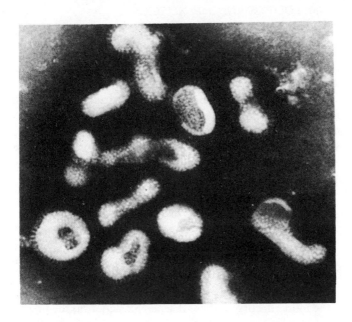

Figure 6. Electron microscope picture of the influenza virus, magnified 200,000 times. (Reproduced with permission from Beveridge, *Influenza: The Last Great Plague.*)

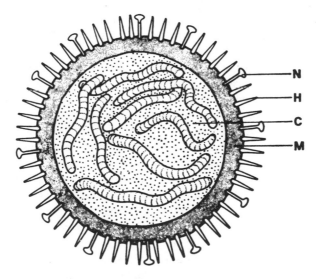

Diagram of a section through influenza virus.
N = Neuraminidase, H = Haemagglutinin,
C = Core containing genes and protein, M = Membrane
   I.—6

Figure 7. Diagrammatic representation of the influenza virus. (Reproduced with permission from Beveridge, *Influenza: The Last Great Plague.*)

51

enables the virus to bind to the surface of the target cell slated for infection. Only when bound can the virus "inject" the contents of its core into the host cell, thus permitting the genes of the virus to take over the production line of the host cell and divert it to new virus formation. It is at this stage that the neuraminidase is thought to function, since it appears to be important in effecting the release of new virus from the infected cells, thus helping the infection to spread. In addition, as we shall see below, hemagglutinin and neuraminidase are the keys to influenza immunity.

Immunology of Influenza

When the body is exposed to foreign disease agents, whether viruses or bacteria, it is able to mobilize an impressive array of defense mechanisms to help cure the disease and to prevent future recurrences. Among the most effective of these defensive reactions is the production of specialized proteins called *antibodies,* which can neutralize toxic substances and viruses and immobilize or even kill dangerous bacteria. The substances that stimulate the formation of these antibodies, and with which they can interact specifically, are called *antigens.* For reasons that are not well understood, protective immunity to some disease agents, such as smallpox, measles, and mumps, may last for a lifetime. Against other agents, including influenza and tetanus, immunity is relatively short-lived and sooner or later diminishes, so that it must occasionally be restored to full strength by means of booster immunizations. In some diseases, such as cholera, staphylococcal infections, or the familiar cold sores due to herpes virus, protective immunity seems to function only weakly, if at all.

When an individual catches influenza, or is vaccinated against the disease, specific antibodies are formed against the various antigenic constituents of the influenza virus.[28] It has been found that antibodies against the core proteins of the virus are ineffective in preventing subsequent influenza infection. However, antibodies directed against the hemagglutinin (H antigen) are extremely effective, since they interfere with the first stage of penetration of the virus into the host cell. Figure 8 shows just how effective antihemagglutinin antibodies can be in protecting against A/Hong Kong influenza. In a test of volunteers, it was found that 90 percent of subjects with less than six "units" of antihemagglutinin antibody would get sick, but that the infection rate falls sharply with increasing antibody titers, so that substantially the entire population is protected when the blood serum contains over 100 "units" of antibody. Since the antibody response to infection and to influenza vaccines varies considerably from one individual to another, this graph also shows that protection may be

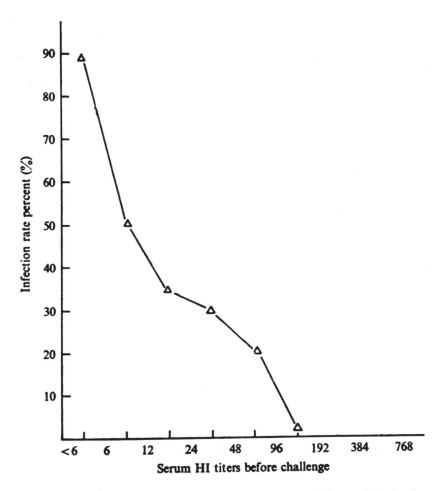

Figure 8. Protection of volunteers from A/Hong Kong influenza infection by specific antihemagglutinin (HI) antibodies. As serum antibody content increases, the infection rate drops sharply. (Adapted from D. Hobson; R. L. Curry; A. J. Beare; and A. Ward-Gardner, "The Role of Serum Hemagglutination-Inhibiting Antibody in Protection against Challenge Infection with Influenza A2 and B Viruses," *Journal of Hygiene* 70 [1972]: 767.)

incomplete; it is for this reason that influenza vaccines do not confer immunity in all recipients, usually varying from a rate of 60 to 80 percent effectiveness.

Whereas the antihemagglutinin antibody may protect the individual from infection and illness, the antineuraminidase antibody carries no such advantage. Rather, by reducing the amount of virus released from infected cells, these antibodies appear to diminish the severity of a given illness, and they may perhaps also interfere with the spread of the virus from one person to another.

One of the principal characteristics of a protective antibody is its specificity for the antigen that induced its formation. Thus, an individual who is immune to measles can hope for no protection against mumps or smallpox, since the protein antigens of these three disease agents are completely different from one another, and there is nothing on the mumps or smallpox organism with which the antimeasles antibody can react. In a similar way, the protection afforded by antibodies against the influenza virus is only valid as long as the same strain of influenza with the same surface antigens appears the next time. Should the surface antigens of the influenza virus change from time to time, as in fact they do, then the value of previous antiinfluenza immunity will be diminished in proportion to the antigenic change in the new virus. This is the crux of the problem in influenza immunity, and the reason why influenza remains with us as the last great plague — because, almost uniquely among disease agents, it is continuously changing its surface hemagglutinin and neuraminidase antigens, rendering ineffectual any earlier immunity derived from prior immunizations or natural infection by other influenza virus strains.

Influenza Types and Subtypes

There are in man three main types of influenza virus, as defined both by their biological activity and by the specificity of their core protein antigens. We will summarily dispose of type C influenza, since this is not a significant factor in human disease, but is, rather, almost a laboratory curiosity. Francis has called it "a virus in search of a disease." [29] Type B influenza is a modestly significant disease agent in man. Since it does not undergo major changes in its surface structure, it tends to be continuously present in endemic form within the population, breaking out only sporadically to produce usually mild epidemics. In most years it contributes slightly to the total influenza/pneumonia death statistic, but even when it spreads in epidemic form, as it has eight times in the last forty-five years, it rarely carries with it the heavy toll in disease or death that characterizes type A influenza.

It is, in fact, type A influenza that causes the greatest worries for public health officials. It is this virus that periodically sweeps the world in pandemic form and, between major pandemics, may break out in various countries as major or minor epidemics, each time exacting a significant excess mortality.

The Changeable Virus

Whenever a major outbreak of type A influenza occurs, it is found that the virus, somewhat like a chameleon, has changed the molecules of its coat. When knowledge developed about the hemagglutinin (H) and neuraminidase (N) surface proteins, it was possible to define serologically the degree of change with great precision. When this had been done, it was found retrospectively that the virus responsible for the 1918 pandemic could be defined as HswN1, scientific shorthand for a swinelike (sw) hemagglutinin antigen (H) and a type 1 neuraminidase antigen (N1). About 1929, a new flu virus appeared which involved a change in the H protein, but not in the N protein: this was identified as H0N1. Subsequently, in 1946, the pandemic was accompanied by a further change in the H protein to H1N1, whereas the major Asian pandemic of 1957 was classified as H2N2, involving a change in both H and N molecules. The pandemic of 1968 involved only a further shift in the hemagglutinin (H3N2).

The new influenza virus that hit Fort Dix in January 1976 also involved a double shift in the H and N antigens, but in this case represented an apparent reversion back to the agent of the 1918 pandemic (HswN1). Among virologists, the informal name of this virus is A/swine, but its full formal name is A/New Jersey/8/76 (Hsw1N1). This standard nomenclature indicates that the virus is type A, identified in New Jersey, from their eighth isolate, in 1976, with the composition of a swine 1 hemagglutinin and group 1 neuraminidase.

The reappearance of a swine influenza virus after an absence of almost fifty years did not surprise the scientific community. During the period of modern virology, only five different H antigens and three different N antigens had been identified on the A virus which causes influenza in humans. If this number were really so limited, then repeated major antigenic shifts might be expected to lead sooner or later to the reappearance of an earlier strain. This idea was strongly reinforced by the observation by medical archaeologists that the blood of very old people had a very curious distribution of antiinfluenza antibodies. Those individuals born before 1889 possessed antibodies specific for the H2 antigen, which only reappeared during the pandemic of Asian influenza in 1957 (H2N2), while people born before the influenza epidemics of 1900 possessed antibodies against the H3 antigen, which did not reappear until the Hong Kong flu pandemic of 1968 (H3N2). These observations led to the theory that the major influenza types *recycle* at intervals that may be determined by the disappearance of protective antibodies from the majority of the population — a process that might take some fifty years or more. With a newly susceptible population, each reappearance of the major new variant should lead to pandemic spread and, in a sense, it seemed almost reasonable to influenza scientists in 1976 that, since almost fifty years had elapsed since its disappearance in 1929–30, it might be swine flu's "turn" in the recurring cycle.

The information available to support the hypothesis of a continuous recycling of influenza A types is illustrated in figure 9. The 1889 pandemic was due to an A2-like virus, which persisted for about ten years. No one knows what influenza type was present to account for various pandemics prior to 1889. In 1900, an A3-like virus appeared, but it is unclear whether this was replaced by any other type in the years before the 1918 pandemic. In 1918 came swine flu (A/sw), and, in sequence, A0 in about 1929, A1 in 1946, A2 again in 1957, and A3 in 1968.

What causes these major alterations in the surface molecules of the influenza virus? Scientists originally thought that these alterations might be due to mutations that affect the individual genes within the core of the virus particle. However, genetic mutations usually impose only slight changes upon the structure of the protein product of that gene, whereas it was quickly observed that the antigenic shifts in the flu virus were accompanied by completely different H or N antigens.[30] This led to the suggestion that the large number of influenza A viruses known to exist in the animal kingdom (most notably among pigs, horses, and birds[31]) might provide a reservoir for the exchange of genetic information with human influenza strains.

The notion that recombinant viruses with new antigenic combinations might result from the mixture of genes from two different viral sources was put to the test in the research laboratory and was quickly demonstrated to be possible. This was accomplished by simultaneously infecting an animal with two completely different flu viruses (see figure 10). When both viruses grow in a single cell, their genes can apparently be mixed in different combinations; some of the viral products will be hybrids able to breed and cause disease on their own. In the example shown, a mixed infection of swine and fowl viruses resulted in the isolation of hybrids, some of which were H/swine N/fowl and some H/fowl and N/swine in antigenic composition. The results suggest the strong likelihood that, while a pure swine virus may be noninfectious or nontransmissible in man, a recombinant virus with swine antigen on its surface and human-type genes that control disease transmission in its core might set the stage for pandemic human disease. How often this recombination of flu viruses takes place in nature and why the recombinant succeeds as a human disease agent are unknown at the present time.

We have seen that the major antigenic shifts responsible for periodic

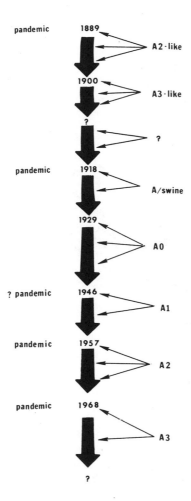

Figure 9. Hypothetical recycling of A2, A3, and A/swine viruses. (Adapted from N. Masurel, *Bulletin of the World Health Association* 41 [1969]: 461. See also N. Masurel and W. M. Marine, "Recycling of Asian and Hong Kong Influenza A Hemagglutinins in Man," in Kilbourne, ed., *The Influenza Viruses and Influenza.*)

pandemics of influenza are probably due to recombinant viruses rather than to genetic mutation. But after the introduction of a new strain of virus, which may sweep through the world in pandemic form for a year or two, it is not uncommon to see milder epidemics follow at two- to three-year intervals for several cycles, until a new recombinant virus replaces the old type, as the Hong Kong virus of 1968 (H3N2) replaced the Asian virus of 1957 (H2N2). A careful study of the viruses responsible for each

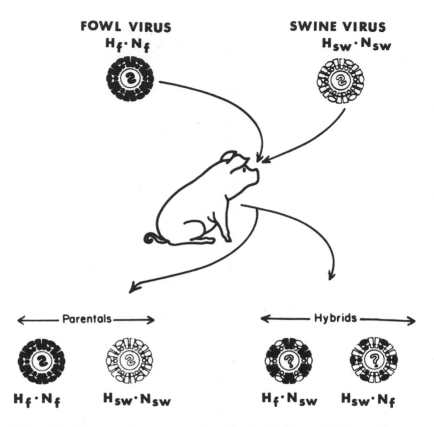

Figure 10. Diagrammatic representation of a mixed influenza infection with two different animal viruses, resulting in the formation of influenza A hybrids with different combinations of H and N antigens on their surface. (Adapted from R. G. Webster, *Current Topics in Microbiology and Immunology* 59 [1972]: 75.)

of these interpandemic recurrences (see figure 5) shows that while they are all related to the original pandemic strain, minor variations in the surface antigens can be seen from one epidemic to the next. These lesser changes are associated with spot mutations in the genes that control the production of the hemagglutinin and/or the neuraminidase antigens. Each such antigenic change means that the new virus is less likely to be neutralized by the protective antibodies developed against the previous strain, so that the new strain will have a competitive advantage for survival and will spread. The further a virus mutates away from its parent strain, the more likely it is to infect those individuals who had, either through infection or by vac-

cination, developed earlier immunity to the parent strain. It is this factor
that keeps the preventive medicine specialists on their toes, since any vaccine employed should be made against the influenza strain *then* in circula-
tion; the appearance of a new mutant would reduce the efficacy of a vaccine made from an earlier strain of virus.

Infectivity and Virulence

The seriousness of a disease in a population is usually measured by
two factors: the total number of people who develop clinical disease, and
the severity of the typical case. The term *communicability* is employed to
describe the ease of spread of disease within a population. It reflects the
sum of a number of different factors, some of which stem from the intrinsic characteristics of the disease agent and some from the susceptibility of
the population at risk. Thus, the communicability of a disease will depend
in part on the ease with which the virus can infect and be released from
host cells, its rate of growth in the infected individual, and its stability
when sneezed out into the air; but equally important to communicability
is the level of immunity within the population at large.

The *severity* of a given case of influenza, and the chance of its leading to
death, is related to all of these factors, as well as to the general health of the
infected individual. That is why elderly or already sick individuals are
normally considered the highest risk group for influenza — because
already-diseased lungs, or a bad heart condition, or general disability
increases the risk of serious complications. In addition to all of these factors, the severity of the disease depends also upon an innate property of
the agent called its *virulence*. For obscure reasons, a bacterial or viral agent
that one year produces a fairly mild disease in the population may, during
another year, produce a very serious disease with a much higher mortality
rate. The swine flu virus which caused the 1918–19 pandemic was
extraordinarily virulent, while the swine flu strains which reappeared
periodically during the 1920s were far less virulent, and caused a much
lower mortality rate.

Even though the scientists have so carefully dissected the influenza
virus that they are able to define precisely its structure and the function of
each of its components, they still do not know what it is about the virus
that contributes to differences in communicability or virulence. Here
again, large gaps in their knowledge made the scientific community
unable to answer the president's question on how serious a swine flu
pandemic would be, if it came.

Vaccines

One of the most impressive medical advances of this century, and perhaps the greatest contributor to our increased life expectancy, has been the conquest of most of the deadly infectious diseases in medically advanced societies. While this was accomplished in part through the introduction of antibiotics and other therapeutic measures, the *prevention* of disease has undoubtedly saved far more lives than the cure. The most important weapon by far in the armamentarium of preventive medicine is the use of specific vaccines to immunize the individual against certain infectious diseases, prior to natural exposure to the disease agent. This approach, through the usually mandatory inoculation of children with DPT vaccines, has made diptheria, pertussis (whooping cough), and tetanus medical rarities in economically advanced societies. Similarly, poliomyelitis has been substantially reduced within the past twenty years, and measles and rubella (German measles) are rapidly disappearing in the face of more widespread use of newly developed vaccines. In 1980 the World Health Organization was able to announce officially the eradication of smallpox, following a world-wide campaign of vaccination.[32]

Preventive vaccines may be prepared in several different ways. In the case of smallpox, immunization is accomplished using the live vaccinia (cowpox) virus which, while not usually a disease agent in the human, will stimulate an immune response that also protects against the related but much more dangerous smallpox virus. Another approach to preventive immunization lies in the use of live but *attenuated* disease agents. As with the Sabin oral polio vaccine, these are special strains of live agents that have lost their disease-causing properties, but retain their ability to stimulate a protective immune response in the immunized host. Finally, a number of different vaccines are prepared from killed viruses or bacteria, such as the Salk polio vaccine that was first introduced in the early 1950s.

There exists to this very day a lively controversy within the scientific and public health communities about the relative merits of killed versus live vaccines, as exemplified by the continuing battle between Jonas Salk and Albert Sabin over their respective polio vaccines. On the one hand, proponents of live vaccines point out that dead vaccines induce lower levels of immunity, and for shorter duration. Proponents of killed vaccines, on the other hand, point out that there is always the danger that the attenuated live vaccine may revert to virulent form and cause disease, and even that some of these avirulent live vaccines may harm the fetus if administered to pregnant women. This argument continues unresolved, with reputable scientists to be found on both sides of the issue.

The same argument about live versus killed vaccines is also involved with respect to preventive immunization against influenza, but in this case it is the dead virus vaccine that has maintained favor among the professionals. This is due in no small measure to the increasing difficulty of obtaining a governmental license, in these times of medical litigation and of increasing regulation of all biological products, for a new live virus vaccine.

The typical influenza vaccine is produced approximately as follows. The appropriate strain of flu virus, containing the desired H and N antigens, and perhaps hybridized with another strain to improve its growth characteristics, is inoculated into embryonated eggs. The virus multiplies, and the virus-rich fluids of the egg are harvested and subjected to a series of purification steps to separate the virus from most of the egg substances. The purified virus is then subjected to a formaldehyde treatment in order to render it noninfectious, and the product is then tested for sterility and potency. Since the influenza virus itself is capable of agglutinating the red blood cells of chickens, the amount of virus in the preparation is measured in terms of chick cell agglutination (CCA) units. The vaccine is then diluted to a standard dosage (for example, 200 or 400 CCA units), and subjected to field trials in human subjecs to assess its *efficacy* (in terms of the adequacy of the immune response in vaccinated individuals) and its *safety* (in terms of the extent of undesired side reactions following vaccination).

The problems of efficacy and safety constantly trouble the flu vaccine planner, and are important in the history of the swine flu immunization campaign. The influenza virus is by its very nature somewhat toxic, giving rise to a significant number of sore arms and fevers within the first day or two after administration. The incidence of these side effects can be lowered by reducing the amount of virus, but this threatens to reduce the ability of the vaccine to elicit the desired immune response. In an effort to get around this problem, several companies introduced the so-called split-virus vaccine, for which the intact virus particle is subjected to chemical treatment and then further purified, in an effort to get rid of toxic substances without losing the desired antigens. To a certain extent this works, but the split-virus vaccine has usually been found to be less antigenic, and is thus generally used only in children who tend to respond with more severe reactions to the whole virus vaccine.

On the whole, however, a reasonable balance can usually be struck between the efficacy of an influenza vaccine and an acceptable level of untoward side effects. Experience in previous years with many different strains of flu virus has thus shown that the dose could generally be adjusted so that some 60 to 90 percent of vaccinated individuals were afforded a reasonable degree of protection, while the incidence of fevers and sore muscles was held down to a low percentage of those vaccinated. Indeed, experience in the five years prior to 1976 showed that of some 70 million flu shots administered, only twenty lawsuits charging harmful side effects were brought against the vaccine manufacturers, of which at least five were found not to be meritorious. Since the largest settlement for the other claims was only $26,000, a new swine flu vaccine appeared to pose no serious problems with respect to either efficacy or safety.

The only difficulties anticipated by those who recommended the swine flu vaccine program involved its scale and timing — the number of doses required in 1976 was ten times the usual quantity, and these would have to be produced and administered on a tighter schedule than before. In the spring of 1976, there was general optimism that this could be accomplished. With the cooperation of the roosters and hens of America, and with a reasonable yield of virus from each embryonated egg, the production schedule could be met. With the full cooperation of both the state and local health officers and the medical and paramedical professions, and with the president of the United States as sponsor, the distribution of vaccine throughout the country and into the arms of 200 million Americans could be accomplished. Given the best of all possible worlds, these optimistic predictions might conceivably have been fulfilled. But somehow, as we shall see, the planners lost sight of the fact that in the real world it is Murphy's Law that usually prevails: IF ANYTHING CAN POSSIBLY GO WRONG, IT PROBABLY WILL.

Recapitulation

We can now put into precise terms what, in March 1976, the influenza scientist felt he had learned from studying the biology of the influenza virus.

1. Because of its genetic makeup, *the influenza A virus is almost unique in its ability to undergo major shifts* in the antigenic protein molecules on its surface, probably owing to the formation of recombinant hybrids between human and animal strains of the virus.

2. *The appearance of a major new strain of virus renders essentially useless any previous immunity* that may have developed from infection or vaccination by earlier strains — the infection can spread unimpeded through the population.

3. In almost every instance of the appearance of a major antigenic shift in the flu virus (usually in the H antigen), and *in every instance of a double antigenic shift* (in both H and N antigens), *a new influenza pandemic has swept the world.* In modern times, such antigenic shifts appeared to be com-

ing with increasing frequency, and recent experience suggested that a cycle of approximately eleven years had been established for the introduction of new pandemic strains of the virus.

4. *Major influenza strains were thought to recycle approximately every sixty to seventy years.* The 1889 pandemic strain reappeared in 1957, and the 1900 strain reappeared in 1968. *The time was approaching when the swine flu strain responsible for the great pandemic of 1918–19 could reasonably be expected to return.*

5. No major antigenic shift had thus far been identified in which the virus had disappeared from the scene, rather than spreading in pandemic form from its initial focus. In all other recorded cases, it had been the old virus that had disappeared from the scene while the new virus spread. *There was no good historical reason to doubt that swine flu had come to stay awhile.*

6. Extensive prior experience with vaccines prepared from many different influenza strains indicated that *a safe and efficacious vaccine could be prepared against the swine flu virus.*

The "laws" of science are only useful in predicting what will *probably* occur, and confidence in the prediction increases only with experience. In any science, just because event A follows event B ten or one hundred times does not prove beyond any doubt that the same thing will happen the next time. In the science of influenza, unfortunately, experience in the relationship between antigenic shifts and pandemics was limited to only a few cases, so that in answer to President Ford's question, the scientist could only say "I *think* that this new swine virus means that a pandemic is on its way"; the scientist was in no position intelligently to put a number on the probability. Moreover, he could say nothing about its possible virulence.

The more impure the science, the more uncertain are the predictions.

CHAPTER 7

Action in the Congress

THE president's announcement of a national swine flu immunization program was reported on Wednesday evening, March 24, on all of the television network evening news reports. Those in Congress who missed the evening news learned about swine flu early the next morning, from the front pages of the *Washington Post* and the *New York Times*. Among health staffers in the Senate and the House of Representatives, two immediate responses could be heard. The first was a groan of self-pity: here was yet another issue to further complicate an already crowded health agenda during the spring and summer of 1976. While the precise details of the president's program would not be known until his message reached Congress, involvement of the various health subcommittees was clearly indicated. Their staffs would have to work overtime to learn about the issues involved, in preparation for subcommittee hearings, legislative action, and the inevitable questions by senators and representatives.

The second response of congressional staffers, wise in the ways of Washington politics, emerged the next morning at the regular 8:00 A.M. coffee meeting of the Senate Health Subcommittee staff, a meeting normally devoted to an informal review of work in progress and to an often irreverent analysis of recent events. Congressional staffers, if they are good, are not only conversant with the technical niceties of the legislative process but also continuously keep their antennae tuned to a number of important political relationships: that of "the Boss" to other members of Congress; of their subcommittee to other subcommittees; of the Senate to the House; and of the Congress to the Executive. This monitoring also takes into account the reelection prospects of all concerned. In the spring of a presidential election year, a congressional staffer would know the current political score and future prospects of the candidates as well as he would know, in the autumn, the statistics of the National Football League teams.

The staffers' response was one of admiration for the political implications of the president's announcement. Apart from the merits of the swine flu program itself, there was agreement that Gerald Ford had done himself no political harm with the swine flu issue. Struggling against a reputation for indecisiveness and weakness, he was now demonstrating decisive leadership in an emergency, with the support of figures of the stature of Jonas Salk and Albert Sabin. Moreover, he had done this on a health issue, a subject that is always popular with the American people. In addition (and somewhat ironically to congressional health staffers), here was a conservative Republican president, known heretofore only for his cuts in health programs, actually upstaging those liberal Democrats who considered themselves "Mr. Health" in Congress — Edward Kennedy in the Senate and Paul Rogers in the House — on a health issue.

The president's announcement of the swine flu program was further analyzed by the Senate Health Subcommittee staff for its implications for the subcommittee and for its chairman, Mr. Kennedy. Obviously, in its role as overseer of the federal health establishment, the subcommittee would have to hold a hearing, the normal mechanism through which Congress formally gathers the information it needs to enact new legislation, or oversees the effects of previous legislation. Next, the subcommittee would probably have to deal with legislation authorizing a swine flu program. The Congress, through its appropriations committees, cannot pass an appropriation for any program that has not previously been authorized by separate legislation. Although the president had hinted that HEW had the necessary authority and needed only the appropriation of money for the swine flu program, the substantive committees of Congress are always jealous of their authorizing prerogatives, and would look closely at such a claim; they do not often permit the Appropriations Committee to "make law" in an appropriations bill.

The analysis of any issue by a politically adept staff will normally include one other item, and this too was covered in the discussions that first morning. It may, somewhat crudely, be put in the form "What's in it for us?" Asking this question does not necessarily imply anything crass or cynical — rather, it reflects the understanding that every issue may carry potentially positive or negative political or progammatic implications for (in order) "the Boss," his subcommittee, the Senate, or the Congress as a whole. In this particular instance, the president was clearly out front on the issue, and, for the moment, nothing more seemed to be implied politically for either Mr. Kennedy or Mr. Rogers.

On the programmatic side, however, the president's call for a swine flu immunization campaign was felt to offer interesting possibilities. For many years, Senators Kennedy and Javits in the Senate and, in the House, Congressman Rogers and his subcommittee's ranking minority member, Dr. Tim Lee Carter of Kentucky, had been very interested in

CDC's preventive medicine immunization program, and were worried by the declining proportion of American children who were covered by DPT, polio, and measles immunizations. They had fought strenuously to increase the budget for these programs, in the face of opposition and repeated budget cuts under the Nixon and Ford administrations. Now, with the president publicly sponsoring a national influenza immunization program, how could he possibly continue to pinch pennies when asked for additional support for an expanded program of childhood immunizations? Here was a positive and attractive answer to the question "What's in it for us?" which would be well worth pursuing in the context of the swine flu issue.

The first order of business was to find out as rapidly as possible what had already happened and what was likely to happen with respect to swine flu. This involved several hectic days on the telephone by health staffers on both sides of Capitol Hill. The answers (insofar as they were known) were not difficult to obtain. A congressional staffer has little difficulty in gaining access to the assistant secretary for Health, to the director of the Bureau of Biologics or CDC, to the chief army epidemiologist, or to the vice-president for production of a major pharmaceutical corporation when he says "I'm calling for Senator Kennedy (Congressman Rogers), who wants to know . . ." Most outeroffice secretaries have standing instructions to put such calls through without delay. It was thus possible to put together fairly rapidly a picture of what had occurred at Fort Dix and subsequently at CDC and within the scientific community.

Moreover, as often occurs in such situations, additional information began to arrive from a variety of other sources. The Massachusetts State Health Department might call directly, while Senator Williams's health staffer came with information and complaints about the program from health professional constituents in New Jersey. Again, lobbyists for the Pharmaceutical Manufacturers Association, a manufacturer of jet guns used for rapid immunization, representatives of the American Nurses Association, and numerous other interested parties would soon be heard from. Putting all of this information together, the staff could soon prepare a briefing memorandum for the chairman that included the following points:

1. Swine flu, similar to the 1918 variety, broke out in Fort Dix.

2. The president has announced a national immunization campaign and is sending up to the Hill a request for a supplemental appropriation of $135 million. It is not yet clear whether authorization will be required, but we should hold a hearing.

3. Scientists are not sure of the probability, or possible severity, of an epidemic, but an immunization program looks O.K.

4. Early signs suggest that there may be serious technical difficulties in immunizing the entire population by the September-October deadline set by the president.

5. This looks like a good opportunity to press for more money and activity on CDC's childhood immunization programs.

A Kennedy or a Rogers would immediately understand all of the implications of this brief note.

The president did not delay long in sending a message to Congress, asking for a supplemental appropriation to cover the costs of the proposed immunization program. In this message, the administration claimed to have full previous authority from Congress to mount the program, citing various sections of the existing law governing the U.S. Public Health Service. It was clear that Congress would have to act rapidly in response to the president's public announcement: a presidential charge of congressional irresponsibility in the face of a health emergency would be politically unbearable.

The manner in which Congress met the president's request was curious in many respects and reveals a great deal about the differences between the Senate and the House of Representatives and about the differences in style and personality of the members of Congress involved. First, there was the question of authorization versus appropriation. If the president really had full legal authority under the Public Health Service Act, then only an appropriation would be required, involving the Health Appropriations Subcommittees of the House and the Senate. If, however, this authority was contested by Chairman Rogers of the Health Authorizing Subcommittee of the House or by Chairman Kennedy of the Health Authorizing Subcommittee of the Senate, then the leadership in the two chambers would probably bow to their wishes and hold back the appropriations bill until an authorizing bill had passed the Congress.

This led, in the House of Representatives, to an almost unseemly race between the appropriations committee and the authorizing committee to bring their respective bills to the floor of the House for a vote. The flamboyant Daniel Flood, chairman of the House Health Appropriations Subcommittee, wanted full credit for responding rapidly to the president's appeal on behalf of the health of the American people, and he naturally agreed that the president had all of the authority required. But the quieter Chairman Rogers, of the House Health Authorization Subcommittee, widely respected as a sound and conscientious overseer of the nation's health establishment, questioned this authority: he did not think it proper for HEW to embark on a novel and important program whose authority his subcommittee had not clearly established and over whose operation it could not exercise the close oversight that specific legislation would justify.

In this competition for preeminence in the House, both subcommittees proceeded independently with their own legislative proposals, with little or no communication between the two. (This is typical of the many reasons that led Peter Finley Dunne's Mr. Dooley to say, "Th' dimmycratic party ain't on speakin' terms with itsilf.")

In the Senate, the situation was quite different. Chairman Magnuson of the Senate Health Appropriations Subcommittee had always been secure in his role in the nation's health picture, and he felt no need to contest minor victories with Chairman Kennedy of the Senate Health Authorizing Subcommittee. Thus, one of Magnuson's health staffers felt free to phone the Kennedy staff to ask what they planned to do about swine flu, so that Magnuson would know how and when to act. Since Kennedy normally viewed himself as the "big picture" health specialist (in contrast to Paul Rogers, the fine-point "technician"), the staff felt free to tell Magnuson that he should hold off for a few days until Kennedy decided whether or not to press for authorization. The Kennedy people would first test the waters a bit more, before letting "the Boss" jump in with both feet.

The second interesting aspect concerned the timing of activities of the several subcommittees. At the moment swine flu was a hot news item, and both press and television would give broad coverage to the congressional activity. But with four subcommittees likely to hold hearings, the stories would become repetitious, and media coverage would fall off rapidly after the first hearing. Since most politicians thrive on the presence of television cameras and reporters, something of a race developed to see who could hold the first hearing. As it worked out, Chairman Flood scheduled his swine flu hearing for Wednesday, March 30, and Chairman Rogers for Thursday, March 31. When this information became known on the Senate side, the Kennedy staff made every effort to schedule their hearing for March 29, but, due to a conflict, they could obtain their hearing room no earlier than April 1. This was a disappointment, since it was clear that the news media would pay little attention to a third repeat of the same news item, and Senator Kennedy had some points that he wanted the media to hear.

It was therefore decided that Kennedy would take advantage of the congressional courtesy that permits a member of Congress to testify and take precedence over administration and public witnesses. Since it was unthinkable that he should grace Congressman Flood's hearing by his presence, arrangements were made for Kennedy to appear as first witness at the Rogers subcommittee hearing. There, in his best statesmanlike manner, he offered to cooperate with Chairman Rogers in meeting this important threat to the health of the American people, and then delivered his real message: even if a swine flu pandemic does not come, let us take advantage of the heightened interest in preventive medicine that it will cause, and help get all American children up-to-date on their immunization schedules, by expanding other federal immunization programs.[33]

The swine flu hearings held before the Rogers and Kennedy Health Subcommittees point up another interesting difference in style between the House and the Senate. The House of Representatives has 435 members, each of whom serves on a very limited number of committees (where most of the actual work of the Congress takes place), so that a Congressman tends to become a specialist in the affairs of his subcommittee and to attend its sessions assiduously. Most members of the Rogers subcommittee did indeed attend, and participated in the colloquy at the swine flu hearing. The Senate, on the other hand, has only 100 members, each of whom is assigned to a large number of disparate subcommittees. This dilution of effort, plus the fact that a Senator considers himself to be the representative of a far wider constituency than does a Congressman, causes the Senator to become more of a generalist than a specialist, with more demands made upon his time. In consequence, many members of the Kennedy Health Subcommittee did not attend the swine flu hearings, or only put in a brief appearance.

Due in part to this difference between House and Senate, but also because of differences in the personalities of Rogers and Kennedy, the two subcommittees operated quite differently. Chairman Rogers always sought a broad consensus among the members of his subcommittee before acting on a measure, and the Rogers staff served not only the chairman but all the members of the subcommittee, providing them with briefing papers and background material. In the Senate, in contrast, Kennedy usually went his own way on most health issues, often needing only the support of Republican Senator Jacob Javits to assure the success of his legislative proposals; other members of the Kennedy subcommittee were usually content to permit these two senators to call the tune. In addition, there was never any question about whom the staff of the Senate Health Subcommittee served — they worked for Chairman Kennedy, and any other senator wanting extensive information or a piece of the action on a health issue would have to depend upon his own personal staff for support.

In his opening statement at the House swine flu hearing, Congressman Rogers explained the purpose. Swine flu presented a very serious problem, because it could appear in such magnitude as to represent a "clear and present threat to our citizens." He reviewed the history of swine flu, in terms of its severity and social costs, and concluded that the president's request for $135 million represented "a wise investment in preventive medicine."[34] In the opening statement at his hearing two days later, Senator Kennedy noted "that there is nothing more frightening to a society than an epidemic." [35] He renewed his call to utilize the unparalleled opportunities presented by the swine flu program to improve the nation's health in other ways. Would it not be possible, he asked, to immunize those children who lacked needed protection against other diseases while they are standing in line waiting for their flu shots? He would return repeatedly to this issue, until he was finally convinced by Assistant Secretary for Health Cooper that the logistics of the swine flu program were so complicated that any diversion might threaten its success.

At each of the hearings, Cooper, flanked by his many health experts, presented the president's program. Choosing their words carefully, they admitted that there was "a good likelihood" that the Fort Dix virus might result in an epidemic, and while it was very "similar" to the 1918 strain, they could not conclude that it would be just as contagious or virulent. But the threat was there, the means to meet it existed, and prudence dictated that they act. Cooper repeated the president's call for a program to vaccinate all Americans prior to the onset of the flu season. In both the House and the Senate, most questions concerned logistics: Can it be done, and how quickly? Will the vaccine be safe and efficacious? Will they have the cooperation of the state and local health officials, and of the medical and paramedical professions? When pressed on the technical difficulties involved, Assistant Secretary Cooper kept repeating the immunization and timing targets announced originally by the president: the entire population (or at least 95 percent) immunized by early autumn. An assistant secretary could hardly gainsay the president of the United States.

At none of the hearings were serious objections raised by members of Congress regarding the principles of the swine flu immunization program; what politician could afford to oppose it then, and take the risk that an epidemic might later prove him to have voted against the health of the American people? Only a few other voices questioned the program. Consumer advocate Ralph Nader's Health Research Group, claiming that everyone was being overly alarmist, hinted at some sort of federal-scientific plot to waste the taxpayers' money. Liberal Democratic Congressmen Henry Waxman of California and Andrew Maguire of New Jersey implied that a "ripoff" might be in the making and that the vaccine manufacturers might realize huge profits from the program, but it was quickly made clear that the industry would reap little profit from vaccine production. In the face of unknown and even unknowable dangers, there was little question that Congress would respond positively to the president's request.

Mr. Joseph Stettler of the Pharmaceutical Manufacturers Association testified on behalf of the vaccine producers. He told the subcommittees that the companies were already testing the growth potential of swine flu strains, but that it was impossible to predict whether 213 million doses of vaccine could be produced by early October. The industry would, however, do its best. In addition to discussing technical and scientific problems, Stettler alerted Congress to two legal questions that required their attention.

The first and apparently most important concern involved antitrust laws, which might prevent the vaccine manufacturers from meeting together to exchange information on vaccine research and testing, to discuss methods of production and formulation, and to allocate production quotas. Some form of exemption might be required.

The second issue concerned product liability — whether the manufacturers, who were quite willing to be responsible for producing a quality vaccine, might also be held responsible for any side-effects that might occur. The manufacturer normally assumes responsibility for the information on usage and potential risks that accompanies the vaccines and drugs that they produce. Now the government would take over the distribution of the vaccine itself, and prepare whatever notices or warnings might be necessary. A recent legal decision had held a manufacturer liable for an alleged injury in a community immunization program, even though the company had only supplied the vaccine and had not itself supervised the program. The court decision held that even though the quality of the vaccine was not itself in question, the company should have advised each vaccine recipient of the potential harm that might accompany the immunization, so that an appropriate "informed consent" might be obtained.

The Pharmaceutical Manufacturers Association suggested that the government might indemnify or provide immunity to the vaccine producers against an "exaggerated interpretation of their responsibility in any mass inoculation program, especially one of the size and dimensions contemplated." These legal questions were not taken seriously during the congressional hearings, especially when Cooper and HEW lawyers indicated that the problems were not serious, and could probably be settled easily by writing appropriate language into the contracts between the government and the vaccine producers. Congress was later to regret that it had not paid closer attention to these legal issues.

Congress acted with unaccustomed speed in response to President Ford's swine flu request. Immediately after its hearing, Chairman Flood's House Appropriations Subcommittee unanimously approved House Joint Resolution 890, granting the president's supplemental request for $135 million. On April 2, the full Appropriations Committee approved the measure, and reported it to the House of Representatives for action on April 5, with a statement that "a potential health emergency exists which warrants immediate federal aid and assistance." [36] Meanwhile, not to be outdone, Chairman Rogers, of the House Health Authorizing Subcommittee, took his own bill (HR 13012) quickly through his subcommittee and to the floor of the House on April 5, employing his own considerable personal prestige to bypass the parent Interstate and Foreign Commerce Committee by obtaining a "special rule" from the House leadership. Debate on the two bills was perfunctory: [37] the Rogers authorization bill passed by a voice vote, and then the Flood appropriation bill was approved by the House of Representatives by a vote of 354 to 12.

Having passed the House, the two bills were sent over to the Senate where, according to custom, they were referred by the parliamentarian to the committees with appropriate jurisdiction — the Flood bill to Magnuson's Health Appropriations Subcommittee, and the Rogers bill to Kennedy's Health Authorizing Subcommittee. By this time, however, the Kennedy staff had sufficiently explored the problem so that it could present the Senator with a summary along these lines:

1. The swine flu immunization program appears reasonable in view of the unpredictable nature of the threat (and in any event, even if there were good reason to oppose the program, there is no way politically to do so).

2. It looks as if the program will have tremendous technical problems in achieving its targets, and it may be in serious difficulty by autumn, when and if an epidemic comes. Paul Rogers has sent over an authorizing bill, but we feel that it would be unwise to lend your name to a program with these potential problems. Failure to authorize will not really matter, since the president claims authority; if we do not challenge this, no one else will.

3. Recommend that the Senate not authorize the program and that we tell Maggie [Senator Magnuson] to go ahead with the appropriation.

Thus, the Senate did not act upon Chairman Rogers's authorization bill, and Senator Magnuson went ahead with his hearings on swine flu on April 6 and had the Senate Appropriations Committee approve House Joint Resolution 890 on April 8. But the normal political process was also functioning in the Senate Appropriations Committee. Here was a bill that the president had said he wanted badly, and the familiar question was asked, "What else can we accomplish, while giving the president what he wants and needs?" The answer was additional funding for federal support of a jobs program, which the liberal Democrats had been attempting for some time to foist upon an unwilling Republican administration. It was felt that the president would be unwilling to veto his swine flu program just because it contained funds for an employment program, so when the measure emerged from the Appropriations Committee it contained a $1.8

billion employment program as a rider on a $135 million swine flu program! (By the time the political dust settled, the bill that the president finally signed as Public Law 94-266 contained not only the swine flu appropriation but also $300 million in funds for the Environmental Protection Agency for federal water pollution control, and $528 million for comprehensive manpower assistance, $1.2 billion for temporary employment assistance, and $55.9 million to the Department of Labor for community service employment for older Americans. A copy of this law is included in Appendix B.)

When Senator Magnuson brought the swine flu appropriation to the floor of the Senate, he pointed out that no one knows for sure whether the so-called swine flu would be a real threat. It had, however, killed in 1918. If we are all wrong, he said, then we might have wasted some scarce federal dollars that could have been used in other areas. If we are right, then the funds will "save lives, prevent a great deal of human suffering, and save billions of dollars in medical costs." The ranking Republican member of the Appropriations Committee, Senator Edward Brooke of Massachusetts, also spoke in favor of the bill, saying: "We cannot take a chance with the health of our people."[38]

It is of some interest that the legal question of vaccine manufacturers' liability in the program also arose in the Appropriations Committee, but by this time the manufacturers' fears were suspect. It had just been learned how little litigation had resulted from previous experience with some 70 to 100 million influenza vaccinations, and the industry was generally suspected of trying to perpetrate a flimflam. This was reflected in the committee report accompanying the appropriations bill, which indicated that no federal agency should assume any liability it had not assumed for previous immunization programs.[39] The manufacturers' association objected to this language in a telegram to President Ford.

The Senate floor debate on the swine flu measure provided the occasion for yet another political set-piece. It is always more efficient to push one's favorite measures at the stage of subcommittee or full committee consideration, but those senators who had no seats on the pertinent committee could always bring their propositions to the attention of the Senate (and their constituents) by proposing amendments from the floor to bills that had come up for a vote. On almost any bill involving preventive medicine, one could usually anticipate at some point an amendment by Senator Javits on his favorite topics of venereal disease and sickle cell anemia research, or by Senator Magnuson on water fluoridation and preventive dental care for children (known affectionately to Senate staffers as "Maggie's tooth-fairy amendment"). This time it was the turn of Senator Dale Bumpers of Arkansas, who had developed a keen interest in childhood immunizations, thanks in no small measure to the urging of his wife, a public health nurse. Seconded, as usual, by Senator Birch Bayh of Indiana, he offered an amendment for increased funding for CDC's childhood immunization programs. In addition, Senator Kennedy proposed an amendment to increase the appropriations for additional personnel and resources for the Food and Drug Administration, one of his pet interests.[40] These proposals were, for the most part, merely "for the record": the champion of the cause would take advantage of this forum to express his views for public consumption and then, as often as not, might withdraw the amendment rather than see it voted down. Excerpts of the debate from the *Congressional Record* could later be sent to constituents to show that their senator was busy in their service.

The Senate passed the swine flu appropriations bill on April 9 by a vote of 61 to 7, and on April 12 the House passed the amended bill by a voice vote and sent it on to the president. In signing the bill into law on April 15, President Ford complimented Congress on its prompt action. Now the National Influenza Immunization Program was fully formalized, and both the President and HEW were irrevocably committed to their stated course of action. There could be no turning back. This was reflected in part by the change in tone of the president's statement. On March 24, he had been careful to say that the swine flu virus was "very similar" to the one responsible for the deadly pandemic of 1918–19. Now, three weeks later, in his statement at the signing ceremony he stated that "this virus *was* [my italics] the cause of a pandemic in 1918 and 1919 that resulted in over half-a-million deaths in the United States."[41] Statements like this, and the powerful commitment at this high level, would return to plague the immunization program later.

CHAPTER 8

Organizing the Campaign

A S soon as the president announced the swine flu immunization program on March 24, everyone knew that the die had
been cast; it would not even be necessary to wait for congressional
approval of the funds in order to start mobilizing the forces. Time was of
the essence, and everyone would have to move fast to meet the president's
deadlines and to prepare the nation for the expected onslaught of swine
influenza. Above all, this would require an efficient and effective
organization to assure that all of the elements in this complicated venture
were properly coordinated and made to function smoothly. But, as Assistant Secretary Cooper had told Congress, this immunization campaign
was unprecedented in its size and scope (as well as in its presidential sponsorship). Nowhere in the HEW bureaucracy did an organization exist that
could automatically take over a venture of this magnitude. Somewhat
earlier, Vice-President Rockefeller had suggested that if they really
wanted to inoculate the country rapidly and beat the jet-spread, it would
probably be better to seek the necessary competence among the logistics
officers in the Pentagon rather than in HEW. This suggestion (like most
others that Rockefeller made under the Ford Presidency) was not followed
up.

Administration

In normal years, influenza immunization programs were administered at a fairly low level in HEW. CDC would make recommendations
on vaccine composition, BoB would deal with the manufacturers and test
and certify the vaccines, and NIAID would provide the necessary backup
research and vaccine field trials. Then CDC would supervise distribution
of the vaccine through its programs with state and local health officers.
Through the years, the three organizations had worked well and effectively with one another on these relatively modest programs; now it was
necessary to plan a national program, ten times larger in size, which for

the first time involved the interest and prestige of the president, the secretary of HEW, and his assistant secretary of Health.

When the president involves himself intimately in any program within the bureaucracy, it is certain to be closely monitored by the president's staff, to make certain that his intentions and interests are well served. In the White House, the swine flu program was the responsibility of the Domestic Council's James Cavanaugh, and his health assistant, Spencer Johnson. They realized that the proper expertise to direct the program resided in HEW, and therefore contented themselves with holding several White House briefing sessions on the program, and with the request for periodic status reports from HEW. More importantly, they let it be known that they stood ready to bring the full prestige and power of the White House to bear in helping to solve any problems that might arise. Indeed, as early as March 31, the president signed a memo to all of the executive branch departments, asking their cooperation and support for the immunization program.

Within HEW, organization of the swine flu program threatened to become somewhat more complicated. Secretary Mathews thought of the immunization program as something interesting and worthy of his attention in the midst of the usually uninteresting HEW routine; he felt that the president was looking to him for results. He wanted his own staff to design and participate in the organization, and on March 25 he asked Assistant Secretary Cooper to chair a department-wide coordinating committee for the National Immunization Program, which would meet daily. Cooper, however, felt that this would be an impossible approach. No committee under Mathews's aegis, with the department-wide composition that Mathews desired, and meeting so frequently, could hope to accomplish anything. Cooper was an activist, who liked to travel light and act quickly; he wanted no ponderous committee to get in his way. Moreover, he was assistant secretary for Health, and felt that this public health emergency was *his* problem. Very quickly, therefore, the departmental committee started to meet weekly, and then less frequently, so that Mathews's ambitions to become involved were never satisfied. It would not be appreciated until much later that a price would be paid for circumventing the departmental committee. In HEW, the lawyers in the Office of the General Counsel (OGC) worked for Mathews and not for Cooper. In the frenetic days of April 1976 swine flu was considered to be solely a health problem; in June and July serious legal difficulties would threaten to topple the swine flu program, and only then would the organizers wish that they had brought the lawyers in at an earlier stage.

Cooper's April 9 declaration of control over the swine flu program took the form of an announcement appointing Dr. Delano Meriwether as Cooper's own "Program Manager" of the National Influenza Immunization Program. Under Cooper's general supervision, Meriwether was assigned to coordinate the activities of CDC, BoB, and NIAID; to act as liaison with the Congress and other executive departments; and to serve as the central reference source for publicity and the news media. His appointment was to cause many problems for Cooper and for the program.

The first problem was typically bureaucratic. In Atlanta, CDC's Sencer felt that his was the lead agency in any immunization venture. CDC had been involved more than any other agency in the past, and he had on his staff most of the experts in areas that the program would require — preventive medicine specialists, virologists, epidemiologists, and a Bureau of State Services accustomed to dealing with the American health establishment at the local level. Even while he was putting the finishing touches on his action memorandum in mid-March, Sencer had asked Dr. Donald Millar, director of the Bureau of State Services, to head a planning task force, and on April 2 introduced Millar as the manager of the prospective National Immunization Program at a meeting with state health officials. Thus, Sencer was offended by the title that Cooper had given to Meriwether, feeling that Cooper (who had been trained as a cardiologist) would be better advised to leave the management to experts.

Cooper, on the other hand, felt that the responsibilities were his. Sencer could not, from Atlanta, exercise the necessary control over BoB and NIAID: they were responsible to the assistant secretary. Moreover, how could Sencer deal with the secretary, the White House, Congress, and the public; that was surely Cooper's job.

In addition to the problem with the title of project manager, there was also a problem with the individual assigned to the job. Delano Meriwether was a young, well-trained public health specialist who had earlier been an Olympic-level track star. Though personable and hard-working, he was so low on the bureaucratic ladder that he had difficulty in commanding the obedience and respect of the high-level agency directors whose activities he was supposed to coordinate. Meriwether's position was a difficult one. All of the action was out in the field, at CDC and BoB and NIAID, and information was sometimes slow to reach him in Cooper's office in Washington. Press and television reporters quickly learned that he was a manager in name only, and while everyone gave him high marks for his efforts, they soon went elsewhere for their information. In addition, the agencies whose work he was to coordinate had collaborated efficiently with one another in the past, and felt no need of the efforts of an "outsider." [42]

Logistics

In spite of all of this, organization of the program proceeded fairly smoothly. CDC began to organize the state health officers and representatives of private medicine, explaining the program and preparing them for the immunization campaign which would follow. They asked the local health officials to submit proposals for vaccine distribution and to offer suggestions for the development of informed consent procedures for vaccine recipients. They put together a master chart, outlining all of the things to be done and in what sequence, in order to identify and avoid possible bottlenecks. In addition, they expanded and computerized the surveillance system under Dr. Michael Hattwicke. This group would staff a control center that would monitor the entire country, looking for new outbreaks of swine flu and later tracking the immunization program and looking out for unfavorable vaccine reactions. The center would eventually be staffed around the clock, and take on the appearance of a war room on red alert.

CDC also had some interesting exchanges with farmers and farm organizations during this period. In addition to securing the close cooperation of the poultry experts in the Department of Agriculture, in order to assure the supply of adequate numbers of fertilized eggs for vaccine production, the pig experts were also heard from. Both the farmers who raised pigs and the meat packing industry complained that the name "swine flu" might be bad for their business, and might cause people to think that the pigs were contaminated and to stop eating ham and pork. They asked whether the name of the virus might not be changed to "New Jersey flu." In addition, one of the country's leading experts in animal influenza, Dr. B. C. Easterday, raised the possibility of preparing a swine flu vaccine for administration to the pig population of America. In view of the difficulty of preparing enough vaccine to immunize the human population, the suggestion of including over 100 million pigs in the program did not fall upon receptive ears among the preventive medicine experts at CDC.[43]

Meanwhile, Meyer's Bureau of Biologics was working overtime with the manufacturers to organize production of the vaccine. A fast-growing seed virus had to be provided, an assured supply of tens of millions of fertilized eggs had to be arranged, and preliminary batches of vaccine were needed almost immediately for testing in field trials for efficacy and safety. It was decided that all production of vaccine against the A/Victoria strain of flu virus should cease immediately, in order not to impede the rapid shift of all available facilities to the production of swine flu vaccine. The 30 to 40 million doses of A/Victoria vaccine that had already been produced were to be mixed with swine flu vaccine to provide a "bivalent" vaccine, whose use would be restricted to high-risk individuals.

On March 25, BoB held a workshop to review recent developments, discuss production capabilities, and outline a preliminary approach to vaccine trials. For its part, NIAID mobilized its extensive network of influenza scientists and undertook to organize the most extensive field trial of an influenza vaccine which had ever been held. This would determine how good the vaccines of the different manufacturers were, what dosages would be necessary for use in the national program, and whether any of the vaccines caused extensive or overly severe side-effects.

All in all, the situation looked quite promising in those busy days of April, and optimism increased that the tight deadlines would be met. On April 9, Meyer sent a memorandum to Cooper estimating that manufacturers would be able to begin large-scale production of swine flu vaccine in June, producing 24 to 30 million doses per month based upon an expected yield of two vaccine doses per egg. Less than four weeks later, following one of a series of technical meetings with the manufacturers regarding vaccine production, Meyer estimated that 288 million doses could be available by the end of the year.

This early flow of rosy estimates soon gave way to the inexorable operation of Murphy's law. On June 2, Cooper was forced to announce that one of the four vaccine manufacturers, the Parke-Davis Company, had somehow used the wrong virus in the manufacture of several million doses of vaccine, a setback that threatened to delay the start of the program by four to six weeks. For reasons that have not yet been fully clarified, Parke-Davis somehow obtained, not the swine flu virus isolated from Fort Dix, but the original swine flu virus isolated from pigs by virologist Richard Shope back in the 1930s. While these were both swine viruses, they were different enough antigenically that it was feared that a Shope virus vaccine would not provide adequate immunity against the expected Fort Dix swine flu. These millions of doses would thus have to be discarded, and Parke-Davis had to start up its production lines again with a new seed virus.

The news of this human error was soon followed by the report of an even more severe technical setback to the program. The seed virus and the eggs were refusing to cooperate in meeting production deadlines. Everyone had expected that the manufacturers would be able to extract two doses of vaccine from each infected egg, but in fact they were getting closer to one dose per egg from even the fastest-growing seed viruses. This led the manufacturers to predict, in their first production proposals in mid-June, that they might only be able to provide 80 million doses by October 1, 146 million doses by December 1, and the first modest shipments of finished vaccine might not come until July. This meant that the original timetable, which called for the start of full-scale immunizations in early July and the substantial completion of the program by October, would have to be drastically revised.

Another logistical problem, once the program started, was getting the vaccine into people rapidly. In the past, immunization required the use of a separate syringe and needle for each individual, filling the syringe from a vial, and then injecting the vaccine into the muscle of the arm. Obviously, this was a very slow process. The army had pioneered the development of a jet gun for rapid immunization, in which a small amount of vaccine from a large reservoir could be fired as droplets right through the skin of the recipient. A jet gun operator could go right down a waiting line, and immunize tens of thousands of persons per week. CDC estimated that between one and two thousand jet guns would be required for the swine flu program, and started organizing their manufacture and distribution.

The International Response

The Fort Dix outbreak and the response of public health officials in the United States did not escape the notice of the rest of the world. On April 7-8, the World Health Organization convened a meeting in Geneva to consider the implications of the American findings. The WHO meeting resulted in three recommendations: first, that all countries should increase their surveillance and means of detection of the influenza virus to identify as early as possible a spread of the New Jersey strain; second, that the swine flu virus be added to the current inactivated vaccines for the protection of those at special risk; and third, that all countries that could do so should stockpile a monovalent A/New Jersey/76 virus vaccine; however, the size of such a stockpile was not specified.[44]

Numerous articles appeared in the medical journals around the world, best exemplified by a series of three that appeared in the July 3 issue of the British journal, *Lancet*.[45] In one of these, it was reported that five of six volunteers infected with the swine flu virus had only experienced relatively mild forms of the disease, while the sixth was unaffected, suggesting that this new strain might not be as virulent as had been feared. In another article, the leading influenza expert in Britain, Sir Charles Stuart-Harris, hinted that the Americans were being overly alarmist, and that "it is indeed highly questionable whether the amount of vaccine required for all of those between 20 and 50 years of age should be prepared at the present time for any country, including even the United States, until the shape of things to come can be seen more clearly."

The comments of the foreign experts and the actions of the WHO were quickly seized upon by those in the United States who opposed the National Immunization Program as further proof that everyone here was overreacting. This charge was answered by Delano Meriwether, manager of the federal program. He pointed out that the United States was the only country in the world with the production facilities capable of providing adequate vaccine for its entire population. He implied that even if WHO or individual countries wished to follow the American lead, it would be technically impossible. How, then, could they advise anything other than watchful waiting and a very limited production of swine flu vaccine? No foreign public health official could recommend an extensive immunization program for his country and then confess that sufficient vaccine to support the program was unavailable.

Only the Canadians appeared willing to follow the American lead, and to institute a somewhat more modest immunization program, working through their provincial health departments rather than on a national basis. They would, however, need American vaccine, since they lacked production facilties. When they applied for a share of the limited supply in the United States, American officials were tempted to accede to the request, until it was learned that the Canadians planned to use the first supply for their armed forces and to exclude children from the program. This was felt to be politically unacceptable to the American public, which might yet complain bitterly of inadequate supplies, and the Canadian request was denied.

Vaccine Field Trials

On April 21 HEW called a press conference to announce the beginning of what would be the most extensive field trials of a vaccine in the history of influenza. Under the supervision of NIAID, up to five thousand volunteers would be selected to test the first production batches of vaccine from the four manufacturers. Using a testing design very carefully worked out by the statisticians, the volunteers would be selected to represent all age groups. Each of the different batches of vaccine would be tested at different dosage levels, and the split-virus vaccine would also be tested, especially for young children. In addition, control groups would receive a placebo, in the form of an injection of water, to serve as a baseline against which the extent of side-reactions and the levels of immunity in vaccine recipients could be assessed.

If the tight schedules required by the National Immunization Program were to be observed, the field trials would have to be done quickly. It was partly for this reason that the original plan called for giving only a single dose of vaccine to each recipient, although it is widely recognized that two doses given several weeks apart are much more effective in stimulating immunity, especially in children. But the planners were confident that a single dose would suffice, since previous, more limited trials with other influenza vaccines had shown that a single dose was usually sufficient to stimulate an adequate level of immunity.

The vaccines used would be closely monitored for two types of response. During the first day or two after immunization, close attention would be paid to side-reactions, such as sore arms, fever, headaches, and other symptoms of discomfort. The subjects would then be questioned later, to determine whether there had been any delayed reaction to the immunization. Each of them would be bled some weeks after the immunization, to assess the level of protective antibody in their blood. As we saw in Chapter 6, although the presence of antihemagglutinin antibody is not an absolute guarantee of protection against influenza, the experts felt that an antibody titer of about 40 would afford reasonable protection, whereas a titer of 100 or more would probably be fully protective.

The clinical trials of the swine flu vaccine actually went more smoothly than anyone had dared hope. Exactly two months after starting, most of the results were in, and NIAID called together a workshop of the experts to report and review the results of the trials. It was a gigantic meeting of several hundred people, including CDC's Advisory Committee on Immunization Practices, BoB's Review Panel on Viral and Rickettsial Vaccines, representatives from numerous federal and state health agencies, and even Albert Sabin and Jonas Salk. The press was out in force.

The results of the field trials contained some good news and some bad news.[46] On the positive side, the data suggested that 200 chick cell agglutination (CCA) units of whole virus was highly effective in adults over 24 years of age. This dosage was found to stimulate an antihemagglutinin titer of 40 or more in about 85 percent of recipients in this age group, which was judged to be sufficient to either protect them completely from swine flu or at least to diminish the severity of an attack. Moreover, it was found that the side effects from the vaccine in this age group would be minimal. Although some critics had predicted that as many as 15 to 25 percent of those vaccinated might suffer adverse side effects from a 200 CCA dose (a total of 30 to 50 million people if the entire population were vaccinated), the clinical trials showed that only about 2 percent of adults developed a low-grade fever (less than 102°) or other mild reaction — a rate that was essentially the same as in the control group that had received a nonviral placebo.

The bad news contained in the field trial results came as a blow to the public health experts. Although the efficacy of the vaccine in older adults exceeded their most optimistic predictions, the results in persons under age 24 were far less satisfactory, presumably because these individuals had not been "primed" by extensive previous exposure to related influenza viruses. In young adults between ages 18 and 24, 200 CCA-unit doses provided acceptable antibody levels in only half the recipients, while use of larger doses would result in too high a level of adverse side reactions. It was thus decided to use the 200 CCA-unit dose in the 18- to 24-year-old group, with the possibility that a booster shot might later be recommended for this group.

The biggest problem was presented by the results in younger children, 3 to 10 years of age. None of the vaccines tested provided sufficient protection without causing excessive side reactions. The whole-virus vaccine would induce acceptable levels of protective antibody, but at an unacceptable cost in severe fevers and other systemic reactions. On the other hand, split-virus preparations did not lead to serious side-effects, but neither did they stimulate adequate protective immunity. This lack of response in children was felt to be critical to the success of the entire immunization campaign. Children, after all, are generally considered to be the most important spreaders of influenza, in their schools and camps and elsewhere. More importantly, the public usually associates children directly with vaccines — how seriously would American mothers take the influenza immunization program if it did not include their children? The experts would be forced to expand the vaccine field trials, to try out a two-dose regimen on young children. Meanwhile, Sencer had to confess that the scientists would not know for two more months what to tell the mothers of America.

If it proved necessary to employ two doses per child, then this would threaten the tight schedule for vaccine production and distribution. The original plans were predicated on one dose per recipient; a second booster dose for children would add tens of millions of doses to the already tight schedule. To further complicate matters, the Department of Defense was asking for 400 CCA-unit doses for the military. They were willing to pay the excess price in headaches, nausea, and fevers, for the added insurance that the double dosage would provide. The primary purpose of military immunization programs is to conserve the nation's fighting force rather than to protect individuals, and young soldiers and sailors do not often file malpractice suits. These double doses of vaccine for the military would, however, impose an additional strain on the limited production facilities.

The vaccine field trials produced another disturbing result, which was not discovered until somewhat later. One of the antigens was missing! [47] Although the vaccine stimulated a good immune response to the important hemagglutinin antigen, it produced almost negligible titers of the antineuraminidase antibody. For some reason, this component appeared to be inactivated during the treatment of the virus for vaccine production. While the antihemagglutinin response is widely accepted as being the more important for protection, all of the experts agreed that the vaccine would be more effective if it would activate both antineuraminidase and antihemagglutinin immune responses. Here was yet another setback to be seized upon by the growing group of opponents to the immunization program.

Public Response

When the president announced the National Immunization Program in March, and during most of April, sentiment in the health and scientific communities was almost unanimously in favor of proceeding full speed ahead. Some voices had been raised publicly in opposition, such as that of Dr. Sidney Wolfe of Ralph Nader's Health Research Group, and hints had appeared on television and in the newspapers that the entire program was based on "politics." Dr. Martin Goldfield of the New Jersey Health Department, who had become more vocal in challenging the decision to immunize the country, advocated stockpiling the vaccine. He "went public" with these views on all of the television evening news programs, following CDC's April 2 meeting with state health officers. In general, however, these negative comments had little effect, and an HEW press analysis on April 30 showed that out of 111 newspapers from 60 cities, 88% showed a favorable editorial response to the National Influenza Immunization Program. This was perhaps reinforced by a letter that Assistant Secretary for Health Cooper sent to a large number of newspapers around the country, explaining the immunization program and urging a favorable public response to it.

As time went on, opposition to the program increased in many quarters. Questions about the validity of the immunization program began to appear with increasing frequency on the editorial pages of newspapers. There was the interesting example of the *New York Times,* in whose news pages medical reporter Harold Schmeck provided his customary intelligent and objective coverage, while at the same time its editorial pages mounted a vigorous attack on the program. *Times* editorial writer Harry Schwartz wrote a series of articles attacking governmental involvement in public health in general, and the premises and "politics" of the National Immunization Campaign in particular.[48] He declared that swine influenza probably would not return, that the vaccine was dangerous, and that the government had no business in such a venture. His opposition was so strident that virologist Edwin Kilbourne felt called upon to submit rebuttals,[49] and at one point a group of scientists led by Nobel prize-winning virologist John Enders of Harvard answered Schwartz's criticisms in an open letter to the *Times*.[50]

As is true of most items of current popular interest, the swine flu affair did not escape the notice of cartoonists and of satirists of the American scene. Perhaps the most pungent and witty of these observations appeared in the May 31 issue of *The New Yorker* magazine. It is reproduced here (see Appendix E) in full, not only because it is so well done, but to provide the reader with one aspect of the public's perception of the swine flu program during the spring of 1976.

Opposition to the program was also mounting among some of the scientists. The most notable of these was Albert Sabin, who in March had spoken ardently for the program and had stood beside the president at his announcement. In a speech at the University of Toledo on May 17, Sabin partially recanted. He called upon the government to hold off immunizing the public, and instead to stockpile the vaccine until swine flu actually returned. At this point, two more months had gone by without another confirmed human-to-human transmission of swine flu occurring anywhere in the world, and the Southern Hemisphere was starting its flu season.

A dissident voice also was heard from within the ranks of the Bureau of Biologics. Dr. J. Anthony Morris, a research virologist who for some time had been having other administrative and scientific difficulties with the BoB higher-ups, was arguing vociferously against the swine flu program. He held that the vaccine was dangerous, that flu vaccines in general were ineffective, and that the National Immunization Program was a big waste. Morris's views were not widely shared in the scientific community, where he was seen as something of a crank, but he did attract the attention of the news media.[51]

These various negative signals had their effect, and HEW's press analysis for May showed a drop-off in editorial approval of the program to only 66 percent favorable. The later announcement that Parke-Davis had used the wrong virus in the manufacture of several million doses of vaccine, and especially the news from the field trials that the vaccine was ineffective in children, would have further negative effects upon the public perception of the program.

On the second day of the meeting that considered the field trial results, Sabin insisted that the question of stockpiling of vaccine be put on the agenda. Sabin argued that, as more and more time passed with no new cases of swine flu emerging, it was more sensible to back off from immunizing the public until an actual outbreak occurred. He claimed that this course was supported strongly by the field trial information that suggested that children, the chief spreaders of the disease, might not be immunized at all, or if so, only much later. Moreover, Sabin claimed that with proper preparation the public could be inoculated quickly if the virus reappeared. Cadres of experts and brigades of volunteers could be recruited and trained locally, ready to spring into action as soon as CDC passed the word. Sabin's appeal was strongly supported by the ACIP's Dr. Russell Alexander, who had spoken for stockpiling as early as the mid-March meeting in Atlanta.

Sencer, and his assistant director for operations, Dr. William Foege, argued strongly against the stockpiling option. Citing a CDC staff study, they stated that there would not be enough time to distribute the vaccine from the stockpile once the typical influenza jet-spread had started. In addition, the public health facilities around the nation were in the process of being mobilized, and any commitment to the program developed in the personnel being trained would fall off rapidly if the program was delayed. Program momentum would be hard to restore, and stockpiling would cost additional money. While agreeing that science could make no firm prediction of the likelihood of a pandemic, and that the longer the time before the next swine virus isolation, the less likely would be a sudden major epidemic, the stockpiling study concluded: "But we cannot be sure. Therefore, at present there is no acceptable alternative to a complete and fully committed vaccination program."[52]

Sabin and Alexander were unhappy with this conclusion, and now did not hesitate to make this unhappiness known to the press and television people. In addition to the disquieting news about the ineffectiveness of the vaccine in children, the stockpiling debate was featured broadly in the press and on all three evening television news programs. The fact that Sabin and Alexander "went public," with its resulting negative impact on the immunization program, vexed both scientists and government officials. Within the bureaucracy, from CDC to the assistant secretary's office to the White House, everyone felt betrayed by their former champion, Albert Sabin. Within the scientific community, the feeling was slightly different. In general, scientists like to pretend that Science dispenses absolute truth and can speak to the world with a single clear voice. Now Sabin and Alexander were unforgiveably threatening this monolithic picture. It recalls the plaint of Senator Edmund Muskie of Maine at a congressional hearing, at which various scientists testified on all sides of what he felt should have been a simple scientific question. He expressed the wish to meet a group of "one-armed scientists," who would not qualify every conclusion with "on the one hand . . . and on the other hand. . . ."

These setbacks were soon to seem like only small clouds on the horizon of the National Influenza Immunization Program: it would soon feel the full fury of a storm that originated within the American insurance industry.

CHAPTER 9

The Insurance Problem

T HE swine flu immunization program had been beset by many problems. There was first the scientific problem of the inability to make precise predictions about whether, and in what form, the pandemic would come. There were also the technical problems of assuring the production of over 200 million doses of vaccine within a very few months, and the difficulty of setting up the complicated distribution network that would assure delivery of this vaccine to the waiting public. But no problem was as complicated and time-consuming for the program, and no problem required such a precedent-shattering solution, as that involving the liability insurance coverage of the vaccine manufacturers. Indeed, for a time it appeared to threaten the very life of the National Influenza Immunization Program.

Liability insurance is an arcane business, understood by only a few specialists. Most of us know little more about it than what is conveyed by the premiums we must pay for our automobile insurance or home fire insurance policies. Even more complicated and more controversial are those areas of liability insurance that involve medical malpractice, especially the large area known as product liability. The past two decades have witnessed the rise in the United States of an era of litigation, in which multimillion dollar lawsuits are being filed on behalf of almost every real or imagined harm. With the increase in consumer advocacy and safety testing, product liability has become one of the most critical issues in the country, involving the withdrawal and replacement, or recall and repair, of tens of millions of defective tires, countless articles of clothing and electrical appliances, and hundreds of thousands of automobiles. Indeed, the Ford Motor Company was recently tried on a charge of murder, because the plaintiff claimed that a poorly designed automobile had contributed significantly to a fatal accident.

Manufacturers of all types, and especially those companies in the insurance industry which provided the manufacturers' product liability coverage, had for many years been seeking a way out of the costly maze of litigation, and insurance premiums had been rising at an alarming rate. This was the legal and financial climate in which the president's swine flu immunization program emerged; perhaps it was inevitable that the program would become bogged down in the insurance controversy. Most onlookers felt that the insurance industry was being unreasonable, pointing to the earlier problem-free experience with almost 100 million flu vaccine doses. To this, the industry responded that never before had so large a program been mounted in so short a time, and with presidential sponsorship. It claimed that no basis existed on which to make actuarial predictions about the swine flu immunization program. Some observers suspected that the insurance industry was using the swine flu program, a health emergency declared by the president and confirmed by the Congress, as a hostage toward having the government settle the broader issue of product liability insurance. We may never know the full answer to this charge, but the events of 1976 should provide fertile ground for students of law and of government for many years to come.

The insurance problems of the vaccine manufacturers first became clear in two court decisions, that of *Davis* v. *Wyeth Laboratories, Inc.* in 1968 and *Reyes* v. *Wyeth Laboratories, Inc.*[53] in 1974. In the latter case, an 8-month-old child had developed polio after taking a Sabin live virus vaccine. Despite expert testimony that the Wyeth vaccine had met appropriate safety tests and that the disease was probably not vaccine-related, the finding went against Wyeth. They were held liable for not having issued a proper warning to the vaccinee, even though the vaccine was administered in a public clinic out of the manufacturer's control. A jury awarded $200,000 to the victim, and the award was upheld on appeal all the way to the Supreme Court. This award and its implications worried the vaccine industry.

All through 1975 and into early 1976, a series of meetings was held within the federal health bureaucracy in an attempt to deal with the problem. While it was pointed out several times that there was the "potential for a crisis in vaccine supply and delivery system related to the liability issue," and numerous memoranda passed from agency to agency suggesting that legislation might ultimately be required, there seems to have been no real sense of urgency in the discussions.

Even early in the planning of the swine flu program, the problem was not taken too seriously. When Joseph Stettler of the Pharmaceutical Manufacturers Association (PMA), in his testimony in late March, warned the Congress about legal problems, he appeared to be more concerned about antitrust complications than about liability issues. Some days after this testimony, the assistant secretary for health sent a letter to the PMA indicating that the manufacturers' concerns over liability should be allayed by the government's willingness to assume the duty to warn vaccine recipients of possible complications.

During the entire month of April, and well into May, industry officers raised a number of warning signals, none of which made a significant impression on the federal bureaucracy. As early as April 8, an official of the Federal Insurance Company (Chubb Corporation) advised Merck, one of the four vaccine manufacturers, that it might exclude all indemnity and defense costs connected with claims developing from the swine flu program, and the president of the American Insurance Association told OMB's Lynn that the insurance industry might not insure the manufacturers unless the government stepped in to provide liability protection. On April 13, the president and chairman of Merck wrote to Secretary Mathews (with copies to the White House and to CDC), pointing out that liability was becoming a critical problem. This resulted in serious involvement for the first time of the HEW legal staff, which called a meeting for the following day to discuss, with attorneys from the drug manufacturers, the problems of antitrust and of the government's assumption of the duty to warn vaccine recipients. On May 1, the other three active vaccine manufacturers (Merrell National, Parke-Davis, and Wyeth) received notice from their casualty insurers that their swine flu vaccine coverage might be lifted. Some days later, the Merck lawyers urged HEW to push for indemnification legislation to cover all costs not directly connected with outright negligence on the part of the manufacturers.

Throughout this period, the insurance industry continued its pressure on the government to take them off the liability hook, primarily by threatening to terminate the insurance coverage of the manufacturers. Without insurance, the manufacturers would refuse to release their vaccine, and the entire program would founder. In HEW, both the lawyers and the health officials felt that the insurance industry was bluffing and that everything could be solved by writing into the contracts with the vaccine manufacturers the necessary assurances that the government would undertake to provide adequate warning of vaccine side effects, and obtain appropriate informed consent from all vaccinees. On May 6, St. John Barrett of HEW's Office of General Counsel sent a memorandum to Assistant Secretary Cooper, outlining the situation and advising that the federal government do nothing more than assume the "duty to warn."

It was only on May 21 that things came to a head. On that day, HEW's top lawyer, William Howard Taft III, met with the chief lawyer for Merrell National, former Secretary of State William P. Rogers. Rogers indicated that Merrell would refuse to participate in the swine flu program without the government's assumption of complete insurance liability coverage. The crisis had finally come. As Taft pointed out in a memorandum to Secretary Mathews, the program could not suceed without Merrell's involvement, but neither could the government do more under existing law than write appropriate contract language assuming the duty to warn vaccine recipients. For the government to go any further than this would mean assuming unpredictable future obligations for lawsuits, and this would be illegal. The federal Anti-Deficiency Act made it illegal for any department of government to obligate itself beyond the sum that Congress had appropriated for its functions.

For the federal government to assume liability for the swine flu program, a new law would be required, and the HEW lawyers immediately started to draft legislation. Shortly thereafter, Cooper sent a memo through Secretary Mathews to the White House, to alert them that legislation would be required to assure Merrell's participation in and completion of the immunization program.

The final blow came on June 10, when the casualty insurers notified both Parke-Davis and Merrell National that coverage on the swine flu vaccine would be lifted as of July 1. A few days later, the chairman of the board of Parke-Davis sent telegrams to President Ford, Secretary Mathews, and to the leaders in Congress requesting a legislative solution to the problem. Almost immediately, Assistant Secretary Cooper announced that the administration would ask the Congress to act, and the next day a bill was sent to Capitol Hill requesting legislative relief. The full urgency of the situation was made clear some days later when Leslie Cheek, the Washington representative of the American Insurance Association, informed HEW that no manufacturer would be covered for swine flu vaccine after July 1. The manufacturers claimed that even if the government prepared the best informed-consent document imaginable, the courts might extend the original *Reyes* decision and still hold manufacturers liable in suits involving unforeseen vaccine-induced illness.

The administration's legislative proposal to relieve the manufacturers of liability was coolly received in Congress. Most members still did not take the liability issue seriously, and the feeling was strong that the insurance industry was acting irresponsibly and using the swine flu emergency for some larger nefarious purpose. No one in the Congress wanted to put the government into the insurance business (although a precedent of sorts had already been established in connection with government guarantees of liability for nuclear energy plant accidents), and above all, no one wished to establish a precedent that might affect other federal programs, including those in public health. Was it not the insurance industry's business to assume risks of all sorts? Why should the government permit the insurers to benefit from profitable programs, while refusing to support unprofitable ones (if this were indeed the case with the swine flu vaccine)?

In the House of Representatives, Chairman Paul Rogers of the Health Subcommittee quickly responded by introducing the administration's proposal (HR14409), and he scheduled a hearing on the bill for June 28. He felt it his duty to help find a solution to this impasse involving a program that he had strongly supported two months earlier. At the hearing, members of the Rogers subcommittee were uniformly unsympathetic to the legislative proposal, and several members made it quite clear that they were deeply suspicious of the insurance industry. Even the administration witnesses were not strong in their advocacy, and scarcely hid their feeling that the insurance industry was up to no good. Subcommittee members subjected the industry's spokesman, Leslie Cheek, to some very hard questioning.[54]

In the Senate, the administration's bill was viewed with even less enthusiasm than in the House, and for much the same reasons. Since the Kennedy Health Subcommittee had not acted on the original swine flu legislation two months earlier, they were content to let Paul Rogers in the House wrestle with this difficult problem. Members of Kennedy's and Javits's staffs met together and recommended that the Senate hold off on any action until things were made clearer in the Rogers subcommittee; thus the Senate did not hold a hearing on the administration's bill. (It was about this time that the swine flu issue was named the "tar baby" by Health Subcommittee minority counsel Jay Cutler, after the nursery story character who returned repeatedly to dirty the hands of everyone who touched him.)

The Congress knew little about the intricacies of insurance. The insurance industry is not federally regulated, and indeed the McCarran-Ferguson Anti-trust Act specifically exempts insurance companies from federal regulation. The only previous experience the health subcommittees of Congress had had with insurance companies occurred in an earlier investigation of the growing problem of medical malpractice, and the experience left a bad impression of the insurance industry on most congressmen and senators. When asked for specific information on how they established insurance rates, the industry was often evasive, and the information that was provided was often too complicated to understand. It was then that Congress first realized the full power of the industry to halt any program that they would not insure, and this power was strongly resented.

The Rogers subcommittee made no progress at its June 28 hearing. The insurance industry was adamant in its refusal to underwrite what it claimed was an incalculable risk, without government backing. The manufacturers would not produce and release vaccine without insurance, and Congress was loathe to pass precedent-making legislation that it found financially and politically unpalatable.

In a valiant effort to mediate the situation, Chairman Rogers called an unusual informal meeting on July 1 in his subcommittee's hearing room. This was a gigantic meeting, at which subcommittee members sat in their usual seats on the raised dais, while the largest table available was placed in the well of the hearing room, around which were seated literally scores of insurance industry presidents, vice presidents, and lawyers, pharmaceutical industry executives, and HEW lawyers. Rogers appealed to the patriotism and social conscience of all concerned, and pleaded for a solution to the insurance impasse so that this vital health program could go forward. Several hours were spent, sometimes in heated debate and sometimes in stonewalling silence. At one point, Chairman Rogers attempted to solve the problem by going round the table like an auctioneer, trying to solicit from the insurance company executives bids on whatever portion of the insurance package they each might be willing to cover.[55] This approach was doomed to failure, however, since it reflected a lack of understanding of how the insurance industry functions.

The insurance policy on a major program like this resembles a large layer cake. A single large company might have its name on the policy, but it would only assume responsibility for the first layer of insurance, and then would cut this layer into smaller pieces and distribute these pieces for reinsurance with other companies, spreading the risk while spreading the premium. The next layer of the cake would be similarly divided among a number of other coinsurers, until finally the entire insurance cake might be distributed and subscribed by thirty or forty companies, located all around the world. No executive seated around the table could announce a major subscription without being sure that he would later be able to "lay off" a portion of the risk elsewhere.

Chairman Rogers was finally forced to throw up his hands in despair. He told all concerned that Congress could not pass the administration's indemnification bill, and he asked HEW General Counsel Taft to press the manufacturers and insurers for a contractual solution to the problem, that would not require new legislation.

Spurred by this congressional mandate, and with the knowledge that the White House and the American public were looking over their shoulders, HEW lawyers held meeting after meeting with the vaccine manufacturers until finally, on July 7, it appeared that appropriate contractual language might be agreed upon by both parties. However, the manufacturers insisted that they could not sign the contracts until Justice Department officials approved of their legality and until agreement was obtained from the insurance industry. The Justice Department soon informed Taft that the proposed contractual language would not violate the Anti-Deficiency Act, but the insurance companies vetoed the solution, claiming that it would not solve their own problems.

The great amount of time that was wasted in attempting to solve the insurance problem by writing "appropriate contract language" reflects a very serious failure of communication among all of the parties concerned. From the very beginning of the controversy, the health specialists in HEW, and even their lawyers, were under the impression that the main problem concerned informed consent, and stemmed from the court finding in the *Reyes* case. This view was apparently shared by the pharmaceutical industry — witness their prolonged attempts with HEW to find an appropriate contractual solution. But the insurance industry had been saying something quite different, first hinted at by the PMA's Stettler, but later made more explicit by the American Insurance Institute's Leslie Cheek.

Health specialists, said Cheek, could not understand the difference between a medical risk and liability costs. The doctors understood only that a vaccine-induced injury might result in an award *for justified damages* — the medical risk of harm to the vaccine recipient. But what concerned the insurance industry more, Cheek maintained, was not the valid claims, *but the legal costs of defending against invalid claims.* Others might point to the relatively risk-free prior experience with normal influenza vaccination programs, but the industry was looking at the public's perception of the swine flu program, attended at it was by front-page and television coverage as a national emergency, and with unprecedented presidential and congressional sponsorship. On this basis, the insurance companies felt that they had no way to predict how the public would respond, especially if Murphy's law should apply to this much larger and more accelerated program. They claimed to have visions of many thousands of claims being filed, most of them baseless, but each involving a substantial expediture for investigation, the hiring of defense counsel, and the filing of motions and pleas. They could see potential losses of millions of dollars, even before any award for actual injury was paid.

Even if this argument had been understood, no one in the Congress or in HEW was in a position to judge whether the insurers' arguments were valid, or whether the insurers were merely using swine flu as a wedge to solve the larger problem of product liability. As it was, the message was lost. The insurance industry stood accused, rightly or wrongly, of profiteering from a health emergency and of unjustifiably scuttling the National Influenza Immunization Program.

The insurance problem seemed to be insoluble. On July 15, Merrell notified Cooper that it would not purchase eggs after July 20, thereby stopping all vaccine production. Parke-Davis indicated that it would make a similar decision shortly. Cooper sent a memorandum to the White House reviewing the problems and available options. One possibility was to terminate the program, and another was to limit it, as in normal times, to vaccination of high-risk groups. Cooper rejected both alternatives and instead recommended continuation of the mass immunization program. This was, after all, a presidential program, and the White House should be used to break the deadlock. On July 19, after a meeting with Secretary Mathews, President Ford held a press conference at which he cited the insurance industry for its failure to participate in the program. However, the president seemed to lay the greatest blame at the door of Congress for not passing the needed legislation. He announced that the administration would find a way to carry out the immunization program, "with or without the support of Congress."[56]

Still undaunted, Congressman Rogers and his subcommittee continued their attempts to mediate the problem and held further hearings on July 20 and 23. The insurance executives were castigated by the chairman and by other subcommittee members for not supporting the program, but still no progress was made. At the hearing on July 23, Assistant Secretary Cooper read aloud a letter from President Ford to Chairman Rogers, urging that the Congress rapidly pass the indemnification legislation so that the program could proceed, but the letter had little effect on the subcommittee.[57]

On July 27, the insurance industry offered a final compromise; they would assume full coverage of the first $10 million in costs, and service the next $40 million at a charge to the government of $1.20 for each dollar expended, with the government assuming responsibility for all costs above $50 million. They suggested that if the government was serious in its statement that swine flu insurance claims would be minimal, then $50 million should suffice and the government should accept this offer. HEW, however, would have none of it. They, and Congress as well, felt that it would be politically impossible to justify to the public what appeared to be a gift to the insurance industry of 20 cents on the dollar of claims, whatever the reality of the situation. Finally, on July 30, Mathews informed the White House and Rogers that some alternative legislation was absolutely required to save the program.

The HEW General Counsel thereupon drafted a new bill to be sent to Congress, this time in close consultation with Rogers staffer Dr. Lee Hyde, so that differences might be ironed out in advance. This was a completely different approach than the first legislative suggestion advanced by the administration. The new bill was based upon the federal Tort Claims

Act, which defines how a private citizen can sue the government. It stipulated that all claims arising from the swine flu program must be made against the federal government. It was craftily designed with a number of provisions intended to hold down unmeritorious claims, and especially to discourage avaricious lawyers from talking clients into nonmeritorious suits. It provided, among other things that (1) any claim must be brought against the federal government, whose Justice Department lawyers are known to be tough in defense; (2) the claimant must first exhaust extensive administrative remedies before going to trial, a lengthy procedure specifically designed to discourage law suits; (3) if a trial should prove necessary, it would be held before a judge, who would look to the law, rather than before a jury which might make large awards in response to an emotional appeal; (4) it prohibited the payment of punitive damages (usually the jackpot for trial lawyers) and restricted any award to damages actually suffered; and (5) it limited the legal fees that a lawyer might receive to 25% of any sum awarded at trial and to only 20 percent of any pretrial settlement.

It was obvious that the insurance industry had won its fight with the government. Despite all of the name-calling in Congress, in HEW, and even in the White House, the insurance companies had successfully resisted involvement in the swine flu immunization program. For the first time, they had forced the government of the United States to declare itself ready to insure one of its public health programs. They had accomplished this only because the prestige of the presidency had been put on the line in Ford's initial announcement of the program. Had the program originally been announced at some lower level (by Secretary of HEW Mathews or by Assistant Secretary for Health Cooper), instead of going to the "heroic" effort of trying to save the program by legislating the government into the insurance business, the administration probably would have let the program die in those last days of July.

The president had not yet won his battle. Although congressional staffers had collaborated in writing the bill, it was still the members of Congress who would have to vote upon it, and they were less than enthusiastic. First, they disliked the precedent it set; they were uncomfortable about putting the government into the insurance business. Would this mean that the government would have to underwrite all of its future public health programs? Second, they were unhappy at having been put into this embarrassing position by an intransigent and, some felt, all-too-powerful insurance industry. Third, they hated the thought of making what was essentially an open-ended expenditure of public funds, whose maximum could not be predicted. Finally, four long months had passed since Congress, in its initial frenzied response to the "emergency," had approved the swine flu program. Since then, no case of swine flu had appeared anywhere in the world. Perhaps Albert Sabin and the others were right, and Congress ought to slow down and reevaluate whether the pandemic would actually come.

In this mood, Congress was not likely to enact the president's swine flu indemnification legislation. It would take another national emergency, and the full force of the presidency, to move the Senate and the House of Representatives to action on this issue.

CHAPTER 10

Legionnaires' Disease

T HE Pennsylvania State Convention of the American Legion was held in Philadelphia's Bellevue-Stratford Hotel on July 21-24, 1976. Like most such conventions, it was composed partly of serious business and partly of pranks and cut-ups, and after the meeting the legionnaires returned to their homes in various parts of Pennsylvania, tired but content. It was only late in the following week that some of those who had attended the convention began to feel unwell and sought the care of their doctors, but the early cases were scattered all around the state, and there was no one to receive all of the reports and draw the necessary inferences. Thus, on Friday, July 30, Dr. Ernest Campbell of Bloomsburg in central Pennsylvania thought it strange that three patients would show up with similar symptoms — chest pains, high fever, and lung congestion. That afternoon he called the State Health Department to arrange for laboratory tests, but he was told that nothing could be done until after the weekend. On Saturday, the chief of Communicable Disease Control in Philadelphia received calls at his home about two different patients with severe pneumonia, but this did not appear too odd for a city the size of Philadelphia.

It was not until Monday morning, August 2, that enough of these calls had been received from around the state to show health officials that an epidemic was on hand. By then, the news had trickled in that many more patients had come down with this unexpected pneumonia, and that eight of them had already died. In all, 182 cases of the disease would eventually occur among those at the convention, of whom 29 (almost 1 out of 6) would die. In addition, 39 cases involving 5 deaths occurred in nonlegionnaires who were later shown only to have been in the vicinity of the Bellevue-Stratford.

The Pennsylvania health officials acted quickly in the face of what was threatening to become a dangerous situation. They immediately contacted the Center for Disease Control in Atlanta, which dispatched three members of its Epidemic Intelligence Service (EIS) to begin looking into the outbreak. When nothing immediate was found, more EIS officers were sent to Pennsylvania, until a total of twenty of them would be crisscrossing the state in search of clues about the nature and cause of the disease. At the same time, the news media were alerted to the outbreak, and that very day what was already being called "Legionnaires' Disease" was given great prominence on the front pages of newspapers and on all of the television news reports throughout the country.

It is not at all surprising that upon hearing of this deadly outbreak of disease in Philadelphia, everyone immediately thought that swine flu had returned. With all of the predictions of a return of the Fort Dix influenza, and with all of the talk of a national immunization campaign, this was the first association that a sensitized public would make. Indeed, this conclusion quickly received important support from the pathologists who examined those who had died of the disease. They reported that the pneumonia that had caused the Pennsylvania deaths looked very much like the viral pneumonia associated with severe influenza infection. The specter of another deadly 1918–19 influenza pandemic was again raised in the land.

If swine flu had made 1976 a difficult year for CDC, Legionnaires' Disease made it almost impossible, bringing into question the usefulness of the agency and the competence of its scientists. CDC's principal competence lies in those infectious diseases caused by microbes and viruses; they sent in their team of medical detectives to Philadelphia, confidently expecting them quickly to identify the infectious agent responsible for the outbreak. Within days, it became clear that swine flu virus was not the culprit in Philadelphia. But what was? Week after week and month after month went by, but the CDC scientists were unable to grow and identify any disease agent from the Pennsylvania specimens. Early on, the possibility of a toxic agent was considered, but this was thought highly unlikely. CDC was soon to come under fire for not pursuing this possibility more intently, and for their relative weakness in the specialty of toxicology.

In December of 1976, Congressman John M. Murphy of New York, in the chair of the House Subcommittee on Consumer Protection and Finance, conducted a hearing to find out what was wrong with CDC's investigation. CDC was roundly criticized for not having solved the case, and Murphy declared that "it was totally unacceptable that in a country of 200 million people, supposedly with the most advanced technology in the world, we find ourselves in a position of not knowing what happened in Philadelphia and, even worse, not being in a position to prevent it from happening again."[58] Ultimately, however, CDC would be vindicated when they finally showed that the agent responsible for Legionnaires' Disease was a very unusual bacterium, hitherto unknown to medical science. The epidemiologists were later able to demonstrate that the agent had been around for some time and had caused a number of deaths around the country. Because the bacterium could not be grown using ordinary laboratory culture procedures, it had not previously been identified, and the deaths had been ascribed to other causes.[59]

Congressional Reaction

The frightening message of Legionnaires' Disease, carried on all the front pages on August 2, was not lost upon Congress. In both the Senate and the House of Representatives, there had been little inclination to enact what most felt was an odious and precedent-setting law that would put the federal government into the insurance business, even if failure to do so meant the death of the National Influenza Immunization Program. Legionnaires' Disease changed all of this.

It has often been said that Congress would rather react than act, and seldom has it reacted more quickly than it did to Pennsylvania's deadly epidemic. The administration's new draft of legislation to break the swine flu vaccine insurance deadlock had only that day been sent to Capitol Hill, and little time was wasted introducing it into the House of Representatives (HR 15050) and the Senate (S 3785). Without so much as drawing a breath, Congressman Rogers called his Health Subcommittee together on the following day, to "mark-up" the bill as the first step in its passage. Secretary Mathews came to the subcommittee and told them that there was a "possibility" that swine flu was responsible for the Philadelphia deaths, and he urged a favorable vote. In addition, the Rogers subcommittee was treated to an unusual occurrence. Dr. Lee Hyde, who had been staffing the swine flu legislation for the Rogers subcommittee, and who took very seriously the dangers of a new influenza pandemic, presented an impassioned appeal for the program, repeatedly citing the terrible statistics of the 1918–19 pandemic. In the face of the news from Philadelphia, the subcommittee scarcely needed these additional reminders. Then and there, it approved the administration's bill and sent it up to the full House Commerce Committee for further action.

In the Senate, Chairman Kennedy and his Health Subcommittee responded almost as rapidly as had Chairman Rogers in the House. If this really was swine flu in Pennsylvania, then no politician wanted to be identified as the obstructionist who had impeded the delivery of life-saving vaccine. The Senate Health Subcommittee called a hearing for Thursday, August 5, at which David Sencer testified. By then, however, more information had come in from Pennsylvania, and Sencer was able to tell the senators that while he did not know what the Legionnaires' agent was, it was probably not swine flu. But all of the senators present expressed grave concern about the possibility that the two diseases might indeed be linked, and the subcommittee immediately went into executive session and approved the administration's bill.

It did not take long, however, for the congressional mood to change. Further information from Pennsylvania made it increasingly certain that Legionnaires' Disease was not swine flu. Indeed, the epidemic seemed to be waning, as few new cases were turning up. By the afternoon of August 5, it was clear to everyone that a swine flu emergency did not really exist. If this was true, then there was no need to keep rushing the unappetizing tort claims bill through Congress. After those first few days of excited reaction, the situation quickly reverted to what it had been before Legionnaires' Disease had appeared.

In the House, with passage of the bill no longer a matter of extreme urgency, Rogers was unable even to obtain a quorum within his parent Commerce Committee to consider the bill; members chose to absent themselves rather than vote the bill down in public. For his part, Chairman Kennedy also took note that the emergency was over, and decided that he would not even bring the administration's insurance bill for a vote to the full Labor and Public Welfare Committee of the Senate. Those in HEW who kept their fingers on the pulse of Congress realized immediately that the National Immunization Program was once again in serious trouble, and an urgent call for help was sent out to the White House. Congress was due to recess early the next week for the Republican Convention, and if action was not forthcoming within the next few days, who knew when Congress might once again be moved to act in order to save the swine flu vaccine program? It was now, or probably never.

Gerald Ford heard the plea, and decided to respond to it. It was, after all, *his* program that was at stake, his prestige that would be questioned if swine flu returned that autumn, and it was a program that he still strongly believed in. Now a recalcitrant Congress would feel the full weight of presidential authority, which even a Republican president can bring to bear on a Democratic Congress. The next day, Friday, August 6, President Ford held a press conference. He told the news media: "HEW Secretary Mathews and the leaders of Congress reported to me Wednesday that . . . Congress finally would act yesterday to pass legislation to provide swine flu vaccine to all the American people. Needless to say, I was keenly disappointed to learn last evening that the news from the doctors in Pennsylvania had led to another slow-down in the Congress. I am, frankly, very dumfounded. . . ." Before a bank of television cameras, the president urged Congress to act, castigated them further for their unwillingness to move, and implied that the responsibility for the impending pandemic would be theirs.[60]

This was greater heat than the members of Congress could bear. Here was President Gerald Ford, apparently willing to go before the Republican Convention and into the presidential campaign with accusations that the opposition party cared so little for the health and safety of the American people that they would let this important immunization program die. This would be unbearable during a normal year, but doubly so during an election year.

Since Paul Rogers had exhausted most of his options for passage of the bill in the House of Representatives, any possible action would have to come from the Senate, where Edward Kennedy was the key figure. He did not like the president's bill. It was novel, it set what he felt was a dangerous precedent for government health programs, and he disliked being forced to act in such haste. But even had he decided to disregard the position taken by the president at the press conference, the manner in which he learned about the press conference almost assured that he would act.

As we have seen, Kennedy is an activist in most legislative areas, but especially in health. He always demands of his staff to be kept up-to-date and "out front" on important health measures. Thus it was that he went into a network television interview on swine flu, before news of the president's press conference had reached Capitol Hill. Neither he nor his health staffers were aware of this new development. The first question asked of him at the interview was for his response to the president's accusations against the Congress and, implicitly, against Kennedy himself as "Mr. Health." The senator found himself in a highly embarrassing position of appearing not to know what was going on — one that no politician enjoys. He emerged from the extremely uncomfortable interview furious that the president had put him on the spot, but even more incensed that his staff had permitted him to look foolish in the interview, in less than full command of the situation. Seldom had the staff seen him so angry. He concluded that the situation was impossible, and that the bill must be passed that night.

The normally hectic pace in the Senate was at once transformed into a frenzy of activity. The entire Health Subcommittee, senators and staff, was rapidly mobilized; one staffer was sent to attempt to round up senators for an emergency subcommittee meeting, another to consult the parliamentarian to determine how the bill could be brought to the floor of the Senate, while yet another found a quiet corner in the Senate cloakroom to write the speech that Kennedy would deliver during the coming debate on the bill. Within the next half-hour, Senators Nelson, Eagleton, Hathaway, Javits, and Schweiker of the Health Subcommittee joined Kennedy in a small room just off the Senate floor, for an informal meeting. All agreed that the president meant business and that the Congress would have to respond. By this time, however, word had come in from the parliamentarian that there was no way the bill could be brought to the floor of the Senate that evening. All that could be accomplished was for the Senate to pass a resolution to bring the bill directly to the floor for consideration after the weekend, bypassing the Committee on Labor and Public Welfare. This was done, and the staff received its marching orders; the bill would be considered by the Senate on the following Tuesday, just before recess, and the staff was to work through the weekend with HEW and other legal advisers to make sure that it would be in proper shape for enactment.

Throughout that weekend, Senate staffers worked and reworked the language of the bill, in consultation with lawyers from HEW, the Justice Department, and other branches of government familiar with these exotic legal problems. In addition to generally desiring to make this detested but now necessary piece of legislation as palatable as possible, each senator concerned had special favored provisions that his staffer would attempt to have incorporated in the final bill. Finally, at a marathon session that started early Sunday afternoon and lasted until the early hours of Monday morning, the bill was put into a form more or less acceptable to all.

The bill was cunningly devised (see Appendix C for full text). At long last, Congress would properly authorize the National Influenza Immunization Program. But in doing so, it inserted a provision that prohibited the vaccine manufacturers from realizing any profit on the production of swine flu vaccine. In addition, it required the Secretary of HEW not only to submit periodic reports on the status of the immunization program and on any liability claims that might result from it but also to submit proposals for alternative methods of handling similar liability problems in the future, so that the same unfortunate brouhaha would not recur.

As we have seen, the new legislation was designed to inhibit avaricious attorneys from encouraging clients to file baseless claims. It required that any claim arising from vaccination must be instituted against the federal government. Thus the manufacturers would be free of liability, although the government did reserve the right to recover damages from them if it could be shown that the manufacturers had been negligent, by producing a bad vaccine. This protection against liability was also provided to those who would administer the vaccine — the doctors, nurses, paramedics, and other volunteers who would otherwise have great difficulty in obtaining malpractice or other insurance in connection with the swine flu program.

In addition, the bill required HEW to consult with the prestigious National Commission for the Protection of Human Subjects of Biological and Behavioral Research, to assist in the "development . . . and implementation of a written informed consent form and procedures for assuring that the risks and benefits of the swine flu vaccine are fully explained to each individual to whom such vaccine is to be administered."

When word of the contents of this legislation reached the insurance industry, it was clear that their only remaining function would be to provide coverage for the manufacturers against claims of negligence in the production process. The necessary insurance was quickly subscribed that same day. With the Bureau of Biologics testing each and every lot of vaccine for safety prior to licensing and release to the public, the insurance industry had few fears that negligence might prove an important issue in the future.

The swine flu bill was brought to the floor of the Senate on Tuesday, August 10, under quite extraordinary circumstances. The Senate had completed its main business prior to the recess for the Republican Convention, and many senators had already left Washington. The Senate chamber was nearly empty, and Majority Leader Mansfield was anxious to wind up the session and let the remaining members start for home. However, Paul Rogers had tried once again unsuccessfully to muster a quorum in the House Commerce Committee that morning, and so any action on swine flu was up to the Senate. But if the Senate were to pass the legislation and send it for action to the House (which was also itching to declare a recess), then the Senate bill would have to be in a form that the House could pass without amendment. Rogers therefore did something quite unprecedented. He and his staff man, Lee Hyde, went across the Capitol to the Senate side, where he set up a command post at a large table in the senate antechamber. There, Congressman Rogers and various Senate staffers put the finishing touches on the swine flu legislation, surrounded by a circle of anxious lobbyists who were kept at a respectful distance only with difficulty. Meanwhile, on the floor of the Senate, Jacob Javits (in the absence of Chairman Kennedy, who had been unable to return from Boston because of a flare-up of his old back problem) maintained a polite filibuster to prevent the Senate from recessing. Finally, with the *t*'s crossed and the *i*'s dotted, the bill was rushed into the Senate, where its passage was managed for the Democrats by Chairman Harrison Williams of the Senate Labor and Public Relations Committee, and by Jacob Javits for the Republicans. Through an earlier agreement with Senator Kennedy, Senator McClellan's Appropriations Committee had already had a quick look at the draft, and reported the bill "without prejudice or any specific recommendations."[61] Javits then obtained unanimous consent for the bill to be considered, and it was now in the hands of one of the foremost orators in the Senate.

Javits assured the Senate that the bill was not meant to establish a broad precedent; rather, it was a one-year stopgap measure designed to meet a national emergency. Senator Taft of Ohio hoped aloud that the bill's treatment of the insurance problem would not establish a precedent, and several other senators made short statements.[62] The swine flu bill was then passed by a voice vote, and the Senate recessed with a sigh of relief.

The bill was rushed across the Capitol to the House of Representatives, where there was not even time enough to print copies for the members. According to the rules, the bill could not be brought up for consideration before the full House without the approval of Rogers' parent House Commerce Committee, unless through special action by the House Rules Committee. At this point, President Ford interceded again and called the Speaker of the House, and pressed him for action, pleading "national interest." The speaker then called the chairman of the Rules Committee, who agreed to let the House of Representatives consider the swine flu bill under a no-amendment rule. According to custom, the "rule" had first to be debated and approved by the House before the bill itself could be considered, and the debate was a hot one. Congressman John Dingell of Michigan charged that the House's action was "irresponsible," and that the bill was "an absolute unbridled, total unlimited assumption of responsibility and liability," rather than simple insurance. Congressman Walter Flowers of Alabama also complained about the rush, and suggested that the new law would open the floodgates to lawsuits against the government, while Congressman John Moss of California argued that the House was being stampeded by a national emergency that no longer existed. Paul Rogers bore the brunt of the debate, and again raised the specter of deadly pandemics.[63]

When the question was called on the rule, the motion carried 272 to 76, and the Senate bill was then called up for action, whereupon the debate started again. The principal opponent of the bill was Congressman Waxman of California, who argued that the drug manufacturers and the insurance industry were being let off the hook by this legislation. He suggested that the swine flu legislation was establishing a dangerous precedent, which might in the future be extended to polio and measles vaccines or even to malpractice insurance. "We are being used, Mr. Speaker . . . I think we are making a big mistake." Many members spoke on both sides of the issue, and it was obvious that most of them were uncomfortable with this novel legislation. Finally, the mood of the Congress was summarized by Congressman Bill Frenzel of Minnesota, who agreed that although they might indeed be making a mistake, there really was no other choice. Swine flu might come, and therefore the immunization program was required. There was no time to consider alternatives; the present bill must be supported.[64] When the question was called, the bill was approved by the House of Representatives by a vote of 250 to 83, and the measure was sent to the president for signature, while the House gratefully recessed.

On August 12, flanked by Secretary Mathews, Assistant Secretary Cooper, and Republican congressman Dr. Tim Lee Carter of the House Health Subcommittee, the president signed the "National Swine Flu Immunization Program of 1976" (Public Law 94-380, see Appendix C) in front of a large audience of physicians and media representatives. No Democrats were present — neither the lukewarm Chairman Kennedy of the Senate Health Subcommittee, nor even Chairman Rogers of the House Health Subcommittee, who had struggled so valiantly and long to help enact the president's program.

The National Immunization Program had finally been given the go-ahead, but it was already far behind schedule, and had lost significant momentum. The original plan had been to start immunizing in June, and to cover substantially the entire population by October; now, with production problems, use of the wrong seed virus, poor results from the clinical trials, and the difficult problem of insurance that had just been resolved, it was impossible to predict when the public would get its vaccine. Indeed, immunization could not even start until October 1, because the new law would not take effect until then (congressional budget rules required that this new commitment of funds await the start of the next fiscal year). But perhaps even worse for the program, these events had provided more than adequate time for its opponents to organize themselves, and also had given them more ammunition for their attacks.

Only the strenuous efforts of the president and the Department of Health, Education, and Welfare and its scientific supporters had saved the program from almost certain death. Events in the months to come would cause many to wish they had not worked so hard in July and August to assure its survival.

CHAPTER 11

The National Influenza Immunization Program

T HE two-month delay imposed by the insurance problem exacted a heavy toll on the swine flu program. Vaccine production schedules had suffered, the on-again off-again confusion had seriously undermined the organization of the state and local units that would ultimately administer the vaccine to recipients, and public opinion seemed to be turning away from the program. Postponement of the start of immunization until October 1, as mandated by Congress, did nothing to help the situation. The Gallup poll reported on August 31 that although 93 percent of all Americans were aware of the swime flu program, only 53 percent now intended to take the shots.

When it appeared that the swine flu program might die because of lack of insurance, Merrell National had halted all production of vaccine, and the other three manufacturers had slowed down their own production; none of them wished to have on their shelves tens of millions of doses of vaccine that the government would not or could not buy. With passage of the new swine flu legislation, full production was resumed, but at this point it was not clear to the planners that there would be enough vaccine available for full-scale start of the immunization program, even on October 1.

It was then that CDC committed an unforgivable blunder. Its contract officers, taking note of likely vaccine delivery and immunization schedules, and of the imminence of the coming flu season, worried that they might end up buying more vaccine than they could distribute, thus drawing down upon themselves the ire of an already suspicious Congress. Because of this, telegrams to the manufacturers went out the day after the president signed the legislation, cutting in half (from 100 to 50 million doses) their minimum guarantee of vaccine purchases and setting December 3 as the last day on which they would accept delivery of vaccine. While this might have made sense to the accountants, it made no public relations sense. CDC had somehow forgotten that the president had said "immunize 200 million Americans" and that this was *his* program, not theirs. The manufacturers raised a storm of protest, and finally

Assistant Secretary Cooper was forced to overrule CDC. The deadline for delivery was extended to January 15, by which time nearly 157 million doses would be purchased.

Severe problems also developed on the local level. The original plan had been to commence the vaccination program in mid-July and finish by November. The state and local health agencies had received almost $25 million in grants to assist them in organizing and implementing their local immunization programs. Many of them had completed development of their plans by mid-June, and most called for a two-phase approach. The high-risk groups would be started in mid-July, using private physicians, nursing homes, retirement homes, special clinics for the aged, and local health departments. The second phase, to start in September, would concentrate on the rest of the population, reaching them in schools, factories, nursing and medical facilities, shopping centers, and other places where large groups of people could be reached.

All of this required careful organization, which had already started in some states when the insurance problem arose. Since survival of the swine flu program itself seemed doubtful, many plans had to be postponed or canceled. Even after the insurance legislation had been passed, local health officials hesitated to resume their preparations for fear that insufficient vaccine would be available, meaning yet another aborted start. Many counties that had planned vaccination clinics beginning in mid-September had to cancel them and could only reschedule them as vaccine became available. To compound the problems, no one yet knew when, or even whether, the vaccine would be given to school children, so the original plans to use schools as organized settings for mass immunizations had to be changed.

To help achieve public awareness and to promote demand for vaccine on a national level, CDC planned to work closely with the Advertising Council, Inc., a nonprofit organization representing some of the largest advertising agencies in the country. This plan was also interrupted by the insurance problem, and the council terminated its contract with CDC in July because it feared that it too might be held liable in lawsuits. Once the insurance problem was resolved, a final agreement between CDC and the Advertising Council was still not reached until October 4, after immunization programs had begun. The material prepared by the council was not disseminated to the states and the news media until late November. None of these developments was designed to contribute to the success of the National Immunization Program.

Yet another problem arose to plague the swine flu program. This had to do with the informed consent forms that had earlier so vexed the vaccine manufacturers and their lawyers. In consultation with state and local health officers, CDC prepared and had already sent out to the states some 60 million printed forms, dated July 15, 1976. These were of two types, one for use with the monovalent swine flu vaccine, and the other for use with the bivalent vaccine (A/swine + A/Victoria). These forms (see Appendix D) indicated that the vaccine would protect most people from swine flu during the next flu season, that it could be taken safely during pregnancy, and that "most people have no side effects from the vaccine." The form went on to advise that "tenderness at the site of the shot may occur and last for several days. Some people will also have fever, chills, headache, or muscle aches within the first 48 hours. . . . As with any vaccine or drug, the possibility of severe or potentially fatal reactions exists. However, flu vaccine has rarely been associated with severe or fatal reactions." It mentioned possible age limitations for children, and that those with known allergy to eggs should receive the vaccine only under special medical supervision, those with fever should delay getting vaccinated, and those who had received another type of vaccine during the previous fourteen days should consult a physician. At the bottom of this form was a tear-off section marked REGISTRATION FORM, which the vaccine recipient would sign. It was not entirely clear from this whether the signer was enrolling in the program, acknowledging receipt of the vaccine, or giving a real informed consent to the procedure.

The bill that had passed Congress in early August required HEW to consult with the National Commission for the Protection of Human Subjects on the content of the consent forms. The commission was not happy with the CDC product. They thought, among other things, that the risks and benefits of the vaccine were not well stated, and they wondered, along with some scientists, whether the vaccine had really been shown to be harmless to pregnant women. The CDC appeared willing to accept some of the commission's criticisms, but it ignored others. Moreover, 60 million forms had already been sent out, and CDC was unwilling to recall all of these, for lack of time. Therefore they had printed another form labeled INTRODUCTION, which provided more information and also told the recipient where "persons who believed that they had been injured by this vaccination" could file their claims. This introduction was to be stapled to the original CDC form, and the two-page document was to be distributed to recipients at vaccination centers.

The final consent form (see Appendix D) pleased almost no one. It was not written in simple language, and the two pages were difficult to follow. The instructions regarding children were not explicit, and many people later claimed that it had overstated and confused the case in describing the safety of the vaccine for pregnant women. Moreover, the form was faulted for not having pointed out more clearly the risk of neurologic and other disorders that had occasionally been reported in the past to follow almost any type of vaccination. Not just the consent form itself, but its later use prompted many complaints. There were some clinics in which the form was not even circulated to vaccine recipients, others in which the signature portions were not collected or were lost, and still others in which it was clear that the recipients had not understood the forms at all.[65]

Murphy's law was operating in the swine flu program with a vengeance.

The Pittsburgh Deaths

On October 1, the mass immunization program finally got underway. It started, somewhat slowly, in those areas that had received adequate stocks of vaccine. By the end of the first ten days, over one million Americans had received their shots, and all around the country things were speeding up.

Then, on October 11, three elderly people dropped dead at a clinic in Pittsburgh shortly after receiving their swine flu immunizations. The story broke that evening in the *Pittsburgh Post-Gazette,* in a factual article topped by a headline stating that there was no tie between the vaccine and the deaths. However, United Press International "moved" the story over its wire service that night, and it was picked up by papers around the country. When an article by science reporter Dolores Frederick appeared in the *Pittsburgh Press,* indicating that the three people who had died had all been vaccinated with the same batch of vaccine, and that this batch had been distributed to twelve other clinics in Allegheny County and to cities in twenty other states, the scare was on. Newspapers around the nation ran large headlines, and began to print reports of other deaths elsewhere that seemed to be vaccine-related.

A "body-count" approach began to pervade the news media, and it appeared that yet another plague had descended. Lost in the growing scare was the fact that the three Pittsburgh victims had all had serious heart conditions, and that most of the other victims were elderly or poor medical risks. Despite reassurances from CDC's Sencer and from Assistant Secretary Cooper, the Allegheny County (Pittsburgh) Health Department suspended the swine flu program, an act that was followed almost at once by health departments in nine states: Alaska, Illinois, Louisiana, Maine, New Mexico, Texas, Vermont, Virginia, and Wisconsin. For three days, "swine flu vaccine deaths" were a big story in the press and on the television networks. The national body count continued, and all of the program's opponents were heard from again, now supplied with new ammunition.

The CDC was in disarray. On the one hand, they tried to demonstrate the competence of their surveillance system by releasing their own body count, while on the other, they struggled to convince the country that the deaths were a coincidence and that a certain number of such deaths would normally be expected among the elderly and infirm. Finally, on October 14, the tempest subsided. Cooper presented laboratory reports to the national press that appeared to prove that the vaccine had not caused the Pittsburgh deaths. To reassure an anxious nation, President Ford and his family took their flu shots on national television, Allegheny County and five of the states announced that they would resume the immunization program, and the other four states indicated that they would soon do the same.[66]

It is clear in retrospect that no one could have prevented the Pittsburgh deaths, but it is also clear that blame for their impact must be shared between CDC and the news media. The experts in Atlanta had known all along that any program involving millions of people must inevitably be accompanied by coincidental accidents and even deaths. Indeed, Hattwick's surveillance center had included, among the many possibilities they would look for in connection with the vaccine program, a category called "Temporally Related Deaths." The problem was that no one at CDC had thought to prepare the country for these expected coincidental occurrences. With a little more foresight, the CDC's public relations group might have defused such a situation, by letting the press know in advance that something of this type was likely to happen. In addition, when the story broke, many reporters found it impossible to get through to Atlanta to clarify this very complex event.

On their side, the news media were also at fault. Apart from those few newspapers with competent medical or science reporters, who tended to present the Pittsburgh event in reasonable perspective, most press coverage was unimaginative and superficial — which meant that the public could not obtain a clear picture of what was going on. Only a few were patently sensationalistic, as in one paper that ran a headline "The Scene at the Pennsylvania Death Clinic," describing a 75 year old woman who had "winced at the sting of the hypodermic . . . taken a few feeble steps, then dropped dead."[67]

A later study of news media treatment of the Pittsburgh deaths concluded that the press and television would have benefitted greatly by having more and better trained medical reporters, and that the medical community would also have benefited from a better understanding of how the press works.[68]

Mass Immunization

Despite the wide publicity given the Pittsburgh deaths, and the suspension of the program in some areas, 2.4 million people were immunized with the swine flu vaccine during "Pittsburgh week." As the vaccine became more readily available, and as state and local plans were further worked out in actual practice, the pace of the program picked up speed. Each succeeding week saw more people lining up for their flu shots, so that during the second week of November, 6.4 million doses of vaccine were administered. This, however, was the peak. From mid-November onward, public opinion polls showed a steady downward trend in the number of persons who expressed the intention of getting their shots, in part because those who were most interested had already been immunized, but also in part because of the cumulative effect of all of the negative publicity the program had received. As each additional week went by with no report of another swine flu outbreak, it became more and more difficult to maintain the sense of emergency that would get the populace into the immunization lines. Thus, from mid-November on, the number of immunizations given each week steadily declined, and receded to a figure of 2.3 million for the second week of December.

One of the problems responsible for the fall-off in immunizations involved uncertainty about how the immunization of children and young adults should be handled. It will be recalled that the original clinical trials had shown that a single dose of vaccine was relatively ineffective at ages 3 to 18, and only poorly effective in stimulating immunity in persons between ages 18 and 24. New field trials had been instituted to test the efficacy of a second, booster dose of vaccine, but it was not until November 15 that the CDC's Advisory Committee on Immunization Practices made its final recommendations. The committee advised that healthy individuals between ages 3 and 18 should be given two doses of split-virus vaccine four weeks apart. This announcement about the age group that should have been the central focus of an immunization campaign came almost seven weeks after the program had begun. In the meantime, children and youths had been excluded, along with the opportunity to immunize entire families in a familiar schoolhouse setting. Worse than this, however, was the simultaneous announcement that only some 8 million doses of split vaccine were left in stock. This meant that only 4 million of the estimated *57 million* in this age group could be taken care of — scarcely a reassuring figure for an "emergency," and hardly the basis for setting up immunization lines in all of the schools of the nation.

Another problem was posed by the failure fully to mobilize the private physicians in the United States. It is estimated that only 15 percent of all swine flu immunizations were given by this, the most important of all groups in the health sector. Here again, CDC may be faulted for not having mounted a broader and more effective campaign to inform the private medical community about what was going on, and what specifically was expected of it.

By December 16, some 45,650,199 doses of swine flu vaccine had been administered to the civilian population of the United States, as well as about 2½ million more given to the military and to dependents by the Department of Defense.[69] This was estimated to have covered about 24 percent of the entire eligible population.

The distribution of this vaccine by age group and geographic locality is interesting in several respects. First, as might be expected from the above discussion, children and young people were disproportionately underrepresented in totals. Only 0.5 percent of children under 5 were immunized, and only 1.6 percent of the 5 to 17 year olds received their shots. This disparity reflected the long-standing uncertainty in dosage recommendations for these age groups and the final shortage of split-virus vaccine. The percentages increased among the older age groups, so that the final proportions immunized were 25.3 percent for the 18 to 24 year olds; 30.2 percent for the 25 to 44 year olds; and 34.9 percent for the 45 to 64 year olds. Among persons over 65, which included most of the high-risk group, 44.1 percent were immunized. This was more than double the proportion of high-risk cases that had ever been immunized in a single year.[70]

Perhaps the most interesting results of the immunization program came from the geographic breakdown by states and large cities. Here, the percentage of the population covered varied from just under 12 percent in Louisiana to over 87 percent in Delaware (figure 11). Among the states with the highest coverage, Minnesota had 67 percent, North Dakota 80 percent, Wyoming 77 percent, and South Dakota 62 percent. Places with the lowest coverage included American Samoa at 14 percent, New York City at just under 12 percent, South Carolina at 16 percent, and Massachusetts at 19 percent. But even within a single state, there was appreciable variation from city to city. Thus, in Texas, which averaged 22.6 percent coverage, Houston saw only 10 percent of its population immunized, while San Antonio administered vaccine to over 32 percent of its eligibles. Again, in Pennsylvania, where the total average was 36 percent, Philadelphia, which had suffered Legionnaires' Disease, reached only 23 percent of its population, whereas Pittsburgh (despite its accidental deaths) saw 43 percent immunized.[71]

The great variation in vaccine coverage in the different geographic areas deserves closer scrutiny, since it can tell us something important about how public health programs work in America. Pending more detailed

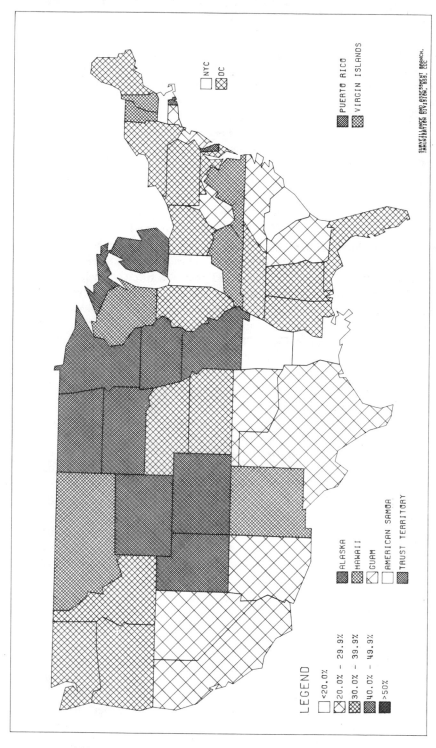

Figure 11. Influenza vaccination coverage by state, as of June 23, 1977. (Courtesy of the Center for Disease Control, Atlanta.)

study by experts, we may hazard two guesses about the significance of these figures. First, we may predict that in the final analysis, the success or failure of the mass immunization program in any area depended less upon what President Ford had announced, or on what CDC or HEW was competent to organize, than upon the commitment of state and local health officers toward the program. In those areas where a positive commitment was present at the local level, effective plans were made. Teams were trained, sites were prepared, and appropriate publicity was undertaken, to make the vaccine available to all who wished it. On the other hand, where local health officials and volunteer groups were unenthusiastic about the program, preparation was minimal or inadequate, so that even a willing public would find it difficult to obtain the vaccine. Indeed, the Commissioner of Health in one state was reported to have advised the public *against* swine flu immunizations on local television. Not unexpectedly, his state reported one of the lowest coverage figures.

The second tentative conclusion that we could draw from these figures is somewhat reassuring. In spite of the generally unfavorable comments about the swine flu immunization campaign that appeared over the course of several months on national network television news programs and on the editorial pages of certain newspapers, such as the *New York Times,* these media are apparently not the strong and unique molders of public opinion that has sometimes been charged. It would appear that the American public made up its mind about the risks and benefits of swine flu immunization employing a broader array of inputs. If they decided on flu shots, they would get them, provided that enthusiastic public health officials had set up convenient and accessible locations. How else can we explain so many states in which 50 to 80 percent of the eligible population was immunized?

By mid-December, it looked as though the worst was over. The American people were, albeit slowly, getting their swine flu shots in the largest program ever mounted in the history of preventive medicine. With the insurance problems, bureaucratic and other politics, and the accidental Pittsburgh deaths behind them, the program managers felt that they had suffered more than their full measure of bad luck and that thenceforth things could only improve. In this, they were to be proved wrong yet again!

CHAPTER 12

Guillain-Barré Syndrome and Moratorium

A LL in all, the tens of millions of doses of swine flu vaccine administered had produced fewer side effects than had been feared. Less than 2 percent of all people vaccinated suffered relatively minor aches and fevers — a very reasonable figure compared with the 1.7 percent of the control group in the field trial who had suffered minor reactions in spite of having received no flu vaccine at all.[72] But there were more serious incidents that accompanied this vast immunization program, beyond the three Pittsburgh deaths and those others that had contributed to the furor of the second week in October. The CDC's program of surveillance made every effort to detect all of these, whether directly traceable to the vaccine or only as a result of a temporally related mischance.

The CDC experts investigated over two thousand reports of serious reactions, involving 181 deaths. Of these, 142 deaths occurred within 48 hours after immunization or involved an immediate postimmunization illness that later resulted in death. Most of those stricken were elderly, with an average age of 68 years. Follow-up studies showed a variety of causes of death, the most common being related to some form of heart disease. In addition, there were scattered reports of various other illnesses, such as adverse effects of other drugs then being taken, choking, motor vehicle accidents, etc. When the statisticians made appropriate adjustments for age, sex, and other medical factors, and compared these numbers with what would be expected in the general population, they concluded that the number of supposed vaccine-related deaths was actually *below* the number of deaths that would have been expected to occur by chance during any given 48-hour period, had vaccination not been given.

Among the many reports that flowed into the CDC's surveillance center by telephone, one came during the third week in November from Minnesota, describing a case of a rare disease called Guillain-Barré (Ge-yan' Bar-ray') Syndrome. This disease developed in a patient not long after he had received his swine flu shot. This report raised few eyebrows at CDC, where apparently isolated cases of almost anything medically imaginable were turning up from various parts of the country. However, during the following week, three more cases of this disease in vaccinees were reported to the Minnesota immunization program officer and relayed by him to the CDC. One of the Minnesota cases was fatal. By this time, three cases of Guillain-Barré Syndrome had turned up in Alabama, and a case in New Jersey. Now the CDC surveillance physicians began to worry about what was going on, and instituted an emergency telephone check with a large number of neurologists all over the country. This quick survey turned up even more cases of the disease, but it was still not yet clear whether these reports portended still another setback for the ill-fated immunization program, or rather represented only another coincidence which could be explained away statistically.

Guillain-Barré Syndrome (GBS) is a fairly rare disease in the United States, afflicting some four thousand to five thousand people each year. It is a paralytic disease, somewhat similar to poliomyelitis, although not usually as severe; in the days when polio was more common (before polio vaccines), GBS was often misdiagnosed as polio. Now that polio has virtually disappeared in the United States, GBS has become the most common cause of paralytic nerve disease.

The disease usually begins with a tingling in the extremities, and weakness in the muscles. This is due to damage to the peripheral nerves in the arms and legs, which may ascend fairly rapidly and involve the central nerves that control breathing and swallowing. The course of the disease is rapid, often reaching its full extent within a week or two; then, over the ensuing weeks or months, most patients fully but slowly recover. About 5 percent of all GBS patients die, mostly due to respiratory problems and a resulting pneumonia, and some 10 percent of the patients are left with a greater or lesser degree of residual paralysis.

Medical scientists still do not know what causes Guillain-Barré Syndrome. For a time it was thought to be a viral disease, but more recently the suggestion has been made that it may be some form of autoallergic reaction to one's own nervous tissue. Whatever its cause, it appears to be triggered nonspecifically by some sort of "health event" in the days or weeks immediately preceding the onset. At least 150 such "health events" leading to GBS have been identified, of which most common appear to be respiratory diseases, gastrointestinal upset, or some other ill-defined infection.

We have already touched on the question of whether the CDC scientists should have recognized GBS as a complication of influenza immunization and warned against it in the consent form (see Note 22). Prior to 1976, GBS was not a reportable disease; therefore, firm information on it was hard to come by. However, the most extensive study of this disease in the medical literature analyzed 1,100 cases of GBS, and found that only one case had any record of a prior influenza vaccination, while four other patients with GBS had earlier been struck by lightning![73] This was scarcely the type of information that would lead an epidemiologist to suspect a relationship between GBS and influenza vaccine.

As additional reports of new GBS cases came in from all over the country, the CDC experts found it increasingly embarrassing that they could not tell with certainty whether the relationship of the disease to swine flu immunization was statistically significant. This was because they had no firm information on the incidence of GBS in the normal population (the so-called data base) with which to compare the GBS reports then coming in. Statisticians can only define an abnormal incidence of a disease by comparing it to what would normally be expected in a given population during a given time, and no one knew what was "normal" for Guillain-Barré Syndrome. The surveillance center therefore sent out word all around the country, alerting doctors to be on the lookout for GBS in both the immunized and nonimmunized groups, and to report their findings immediately to the control center in Atlanta. Only in this way, and more slowly than they would have liked, were they able to figure out the real incidence and true significance of their GBS reports.

By mid-December, CDC had collected reports of 107 cases of GBS, involving six deaths, and additional reports were arriving continuously.[74] But even these very preliminary and scattered figures told the statisticians that the incidence of disease, while low, was greater in vaccinees (one case in 100,000 to 200,000) than in the normal population (one case in more than 1 million). These numbers, although admittedly premature, had to be taken seriously, and Sencer was promptly notified about the findings.

It was immediately clear to Sencer that Guillain-Barré Syndrome probably represented the final unhappy blow to this ill-starred program. He immediately consulted with his normal sources in the Advisory Committee on Immunization Practices and at NIAID and BoB, on the problem posed by Guillain-Barré Syndrome. While many of his advisers felt that the results were still too preliminary to establish an association between flu vaccine and GBS, all recognized at once that the immunization program had reached a crisis. Sensitized by nine agonizing months of unexpected events, of stop-and-go activity, and of crises of confidence, everyone realized that a decision had been forced upon them. Even with only a hint that the swine flu vaccine was causing GBS, there could be no question of continuing to immunize the public. Rather, the immunization program must be halted until such time as additional data might prove *beyond reasonable doubt* that the cases of GBS were coincidental and not due to the vaccine. To continue the program while the data were reevaluated was unthinkable; the program's opponents and the press and television would not permit this, and those responsible for the program would be crucified by the inevitable media descriptions of paralyzed victims in wheel chairs and respirators, and by body counts of the dead.

On December 16, Sencer called Cooper to transmit the bad news. He tracked Cooper down at the White House Staff Mess, where he was having lunch with Cavanaugh; Secretary Mathews happened to be present also, elsewhere in the dining room. The three of them put their heads together, to discuss what should be done, and Cooper instructed the White House switchboard to put in an emergency call to Jonas Salk — the now-familiar appeal to authority to support an inevitable decision. Salk was rapidly traced to Paris where, unenthusiastically, he agreed with the recommendation that the immunization program be suspended. With this information in hand, the group went immediately to see President Ford to apprise him of the new developments.

In view of the continuing absence of swine flu anywhere in the world, and of the clear and present danger to the American people imposed by Guillain-Barré Syndrome, the President could only sigh and concur with the recommendation. There could be no question now of salvaging the program by strenuous White House intervention, as had occurred in the past; the presence of Guillain-Barré Syndrome foreclosed that possibility. Nor did there even exist in December the significant aspect of presidential prestige that had so affected events in July. The swine flu program had not figured prominently (if at all) in the presidential campaign that culminated in the elections of early November, when Gerald Ford lost the presidency to Jimmy Carter. The lame-duck president and his staff had, in December, other things to preoccupy them, and the fate of the swine flu program could now be bequeathed to the new administration.

That afternoon, Cooper announced a moratorium in the swine flu immunization program "in the interest of safety of the public, in the interest of credibility, and in the interest of the practice of good medicine."[75] The giving of flu shots would be suspended while the Guillain-Barré Syndrome data were reevaluated. The option of resuming immunizations was kept open, if further analysis should show that there was no direct relationship between the vaccine and GBS, or especially if pandemic swine flu should in fact appear in the United States.

The National Influenza Immunization Program was, for all practical purposes, dead.

CHAPTER 13

The Immediate Aftermath

S WINE flu did not return to the United States during the winter of 1976–77, nor did it appear anywhere else in the world. Indeed, that particular flu season proved to be one of the mildest on record. The swine flu virus had disappeared as suddenly and mysteriously as it had first come. Apparently it had been unable to compete successfully with the existing A/Victoria strain of virus, and had thus confounded the experts. Of course, had virulent pandemic swine flu actually returned, then the moratorium on the program would have been lifted immediately, and immunizations resumed. Guillain-Barré Syndrome, measured in the hundreds of cases and even accompanied by deaths counted in double figures would have been considered a small price to pay to prevent thousands or tens of thousands of deaths from virulent influenza.

Decisions on almost any medical procedure or therapy, whether public or private, require an evaluation and comparison of the risks and the benefits, insofar as they can be measured. If the benefits outweigh the risks, then the gamble is taken. This is why Sabin live polio vaccine is permitted, although it does result in rare cases of vaccine-induced disease. This is also the reason that smallpox vaccination was practiced for so long — because the occasional case of encephalitis caused by the vaccine was considered a low price for assured protection against smallpox. But once the threat of smallpox was substantially reduced, following the eradication campaign by the World Health Organization, the scientific advisers were quick to recommend cessation of the vaccination program — they now felt that the risks far outweighed the potential benefits.

GBS — Final Conclusions

As additional data on Guillain-Barré Syndrome flowed into the surveillance center at CDC, the picture became clearer, and the conclusion inescapable: the A/swine vaccine was responsible for a statistically significant increase in the incidence of GBS. By March of 1977, 843 cases of GBS had been reported and analyzed.[76] Of these, 427 had occurred in persons immunized with the swine flu vaccine, while 416 cases had occurred in persons who had not received this vaccine. While these numbers may appear at first sight not to be significantly different, each must be divided by the total population involved in order to obtain the true disease incidence. When this was done, the incidence of GBS proved to be 8.3 cases per million vaccinees per month, as compared with 0.7 cases per million of the general population per month. Thus, the "relative risk" of GBS in vaccinees was 12 times greater than the normally expected rate. There were 34 deaths associated with these GBS cases, 17 among persons receiving the swine flu vaccine and 17 among the unvaccinated. Again, when correction is made for the difference in the size of the respective populations, the swine flu vaccine was clearly implicated.

Further analysis of the data reinforced this conclusion. In the normal population, the peak incidence of GBS occurs in the 15-to-19-year-old group, whereas among vaccinees the peak incidence occurred in persons 35 to 44 years of age. Even more convincing was the comparison of the date of onset of GBS in vaccinated and nonvaccinated groups.[77] In the general population, the disease was present at a "normal" frequency prior to the start of the immunization program on October 1, and maintained relatively constant levels throughout the duration of the program. In contrast, the disease tended to affect vaccinees mostly during the first three weeks after immunization, reaching a peak during the third week following the injection and then declining in incidence, so that by nine weeks after vaccination the incidence of GBS had returned to normal levels. In consequence, a graph of GBS cases in the vaccinated population by date of onset of disease revealed a fairly typical "epidemic curve" (figure 12), starting some two weeks after the beginning of the vaccination program in early October, rising gradually to a peak during the week of December 11 (about three weeks after the maximum vaccination rate had been achieved), and then declining abruptly in the weeks following the moratorium.

Although the total number of "excess cases" of Guillain-Barré Syndrome was not large, the results of the analysis implicating the swine flu vaccine were statistically significant. What is especially ironic is that the relationship would have been missed completely had the planners of the National Immunization Program not taken great care in setting up their surveillance system. The influenza vaccine conference of March 21, 1977, concluded that the "risks of influenza vaccine are so low that, had there not been a sensitive special vaccine reaction surveillance system, and had not over 40 million doses of vaccine been given in a two-month period, the

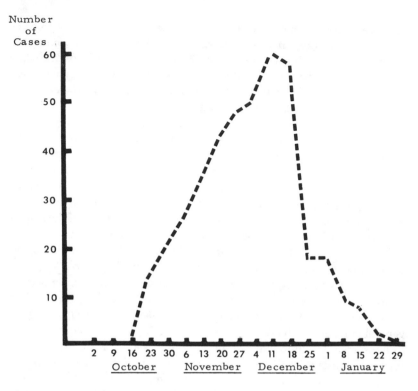

Figure 12. Week of onset of Guillain-Barré Syndrome in vaccinated persons. (Adapted from CDC data, *Summary Report of Conference on Influenza Vaccine Activity for 1977–78,* U.S. Department of Health, Education, and Welfare, March 21, 1978.)

relationship between influenza vaccination and GBS would not have been detected."[78]

Neither the statisticians, nor the epidemiologists, nor other health officials could tell *why* the swine flu vaccine had caused these cases of Guillain-Barré Syndrome. It was clearly not associated with a contaminant introduced during the manufacture of the vaccine, since each of the four manufacturers had employed slightly different procedures and had produced a large number of different batches of vaccine, and the cases of GBS were not restricted to any one manufacturer or any specific lots of vaccine. The scientists thus could not (and still cannot) draw any firm conclusions on the mechanism of production of GBS. However, the attention drawn to this fairly rare disease by the 1976 event has since served to stimulate research on its causes and possible therapy in many medical institutions throughout the country.

The Public Response

Once again, the news media in the United States were full of stories that made it appear that America was in the grip of a new and deadly epidemic, this time the Guillain-Barré Syndrome. Those who had received the swine flu vaccine wondered whether they too might develop the disease, while many others who had not been vaccinated feared that they might "catch the disease" from those who had.

Shortly after hearing the news of Cooper's announcement of the moratorium, Senator Kennedy announced that his Health Subcommittee would hold a hearing on the matter early the very next day. The decision came so suddenly that several of the Kennedy health staffers had to leave the senator's annual Christmas party at his home that evening in order to prepare for the hearing. In his opening statement the next morning, Kennedy emphasized that the main purpose of the hearing was to reassure the American people about the real nature of Guillain-Barré Syndrome. "Hopefully, we will find today, or in the near future, that this illness is not related to the swine flu vaccine. Over 35 million Americans have received the flu shots thus far, and they . . . need to be reassured that their health is not in jeopardy. Fortunately, it looks as though there is no reason for anyone to panic about this limited number of cases reported. I understand from some of the country's leading neurologists that this is an allergic rather than an infectious disease. . . . Thus, it appears that there is no reason for anyone to fear that this Guillain-Barré disease can be transmitted from one person to another." [79]

Neither Kennedy nor other members of the Senate Health Subcommittee raised serious questions about the original decision to undertake the National Immunization Program. They also refrained from any attempt to assign blame either for the program itself or for the difficulties it had encountered, including this latest rare disease that sometimes accompanied immunization. Rather, they carefully led Assistant Secretary Cooper through testimony designed to convince the public that there was no need to panic. In fact, they congratulated Cooper and the program on the surveillance scheme that had permitted early identification of the relationship between vaccination and Guillain-Barré Syndrome. Senator Javits was especially considerate. He stated that

> while other difficulties continued to plague the program, the Public Health Service, under Dr. Cooper's leadership, continued to mount an effective program to combat swine flu. . . . basing it on the best available scientific data which, in the opinion of most influenza experts and public health experts, justified the program as prudent preventive medicine. . . . But as

they made the right decision in March to begin this program, based on available scientific data, so I believe that they made the right decision yesterday to suspend it temporarily. . . . There are those who will say that this program has failed. I am not one of them. I believe that it has succeeded. . . . We have raised the public's awareness of the need to prevent disease from happening.[80]

The press, however, was not as kind to the swine flu program and its governmental sponsors as the senators had been. On television network news, it was hinted that the program had been defective almost from the very start, and now good riddance. This sentiment was made explicit by many who had opposed the program all along and who could now claim to have been vindicated in their opposition. On December 21, *New York Times* editorial writer Harry Schwartz, who had repeatedly inveighed against the program in the past, now deserted the anonymity of the editorial page to write a signed Op-Ed piece that labeled the program a "fiasco." He observed that "the sorry debacle of the swine flu vaccine program provides a fitting endpoint to the misunderstandings and misconceptions that have marked government approaches to health care."

Schwartz went on to point out that:

> Any reasonable effort to assign responsibility for this state of affairs must call attention to at least the following elements:
> (1) the scarcity in the White House and in Congress of officials with sufficient sophistication in medical problems to be able to put biological reality before political expediency. . . .
> (2) the excessive confidence of the government medical bureaucracy and its outside experts in urging the vaccination program on the country while playing down the uncertainties. . . .
> (3) the self-interest of the government health bureaucracy which saw in the swine flu threat the ideal chance to impress the nation. . . .[81]

This was a severe indictment, which would be echoed elsewhere.[82]

After it became clear that Guillain-Barré Syndrome posed no immediate threat beyond what had already occurred, the public was left confused about what had happened, and why. For a time, the public health community feared that the public's confusion and exasperation might translate into future unwillingness to participate in other routine immunization programs, but this fear proved to be groundless. The collective memory in such matters seems to be quite short, and over the next several years public participation in such immunization programs as polio and DPT showed no measurable decrease.

Influenza in 1976–77

With the exception of a very few cases of swine flu that could be shown to have originated in pigs, no human-to-human transmission of the disease occurred during the 1976–77 influenza season. However, small isolated outbreaks of A/Victoria influenza and of type B influenza continued to appear in various parts of the United States and the world. But the only A/Victoria vaccine available had already been mixed with swine vaccine, and could not be administered because of the moratorium instituted on December 16. More embarrassing, it was found that the moratorium had been so worded that *no* flu vaccine could legally be used, not even the presumably innocuous type B vaccine.

On January 14, the Advisory Committee on Immunization Practices met again at CDC in Atlanta. Taking cognizance of the extremely low risk of Guillain-Barré Syndrome among vaccinees, of the continued presence of A/Victoria and B influenza in the population, and of the continuing possibility that swine flu might indeed return that season, the ACIP weighed the risks against the benefits and recommended lifting the moratorium and continuing the immunization program, at least among high-risk groups. Cooper, who also had to add to this equation the public response and political implications of resumption of the immunization program, would have none of it. He had already been informed that his services would no longer be required by President Carter's HEW Secretary-Designate Joseph Califano, who would take office the following week, so he decided to leave this decision to the new administration.

Then, on January 18, an outbreak of A/Victoria influenza occurred in a nursing home in Florida. Of 176 elderly residents, plus staff, 57 came down with influenza and 3 died. Only 3 of 41 vaccinated individuals became ill (7.3 percent), while 56 of 135 unvaccinated persons (42 percent) were struck. All of the deaths were in the unvaccinated group. Clearly something had to be done about this situation.

One of the first actions taken by Califano on entering office was, therefore, to convene a special ad hoc blue-ribbon panel to meet on February 7 to review the moratorium. The panel was a distinguished one, chaired by Dr. John Knowles, President of the Rockefeller Foundation, and with Dr. Ivan Bennett, Jr., Dean of the New York University Medical Center as vice-chairman. It was composed not only of distinguished medical scientists (most of whom had not been involved in the earlier swine flu decisions) but also of representatives from the civilian sector. Since the accusation had been rife that the swine flu policy making had been made by an "in-group," out of the public view, Califano insisted on, and obtained, broad media coverage. After extensive discussion, the committee decided to retain the moratorium on monovalent swine flu vaccine, but to lift the moratorium on the type B vaccine and on the bivalent A/swine-A/Victoria, for use in the high-risk population. The consensus was "that for the elderly or chronically ill, the risk of A/Victoria influenza mortality clearly outweighed the risks of death from GBS." [83]

But the American people had lost all interest in influenza vaccines, at least for the moment. Very few took advantage of the lifting of the moratorium, and of the renewed availability of protective vaccine. Public health experts worried about the implications for the coming flu season of this public unwillingness to obtain protective immunization. On March 21, Secretary Califano convened another distinguished ad hoc committee to consider this problem, this time chaired by Dr. David Rogers, president of the Robert Wood Johnson Foundation, and co-chaired by Dr. James Hirsch, dean of Graduate Studies of the Rockefeller University. This meeting was even larger than the previous one, and included not only an impressive number of participants representing the general public, but broad press and television coverage as well. Califano was determined to do everything in full view, and with broad consensus.

It was agreed by this committee that a continuing program of influenza immunization for high-risk groups and those involved in essential community services should be maintained, and that the federal government should continue its activity in public education and participate in the purchase and delivery of vaccine. The committee concluded that "the federal government should continue its commitment to influenza vaccine research and influenza surveillance. . . . [and] should be involved and should take appropriate action in influenza immunization or the level of immunity within the population will be lowered." [84] Thus, the unhappy experience with the swine flu program did not prove traumatic enough to force the federal government completely out of all future activity concerning influenza vaccines.

Liability for Vaccine Side Effects

The special legislation that had been passed by Congress in August of 1976 made the United States government responsible for all liability claims arising out of the swine flu immunization program. With the widespread publicity that attended the outbreak of vaccine-associated Guillain-Barré Syndrome, and the termination of the immunization program, few citizens (and probably no lawyers) were unaware that the government stood ready to compensate those who had suffered from undue side effects of the vaccine. It was not very long after declaration of the moratorium on the immunization program that claims against the government started coming in. Some of these claims were associated with the development of post immunization Guillain-Barré Syndrome. Some claimants alleged other neurological disorders, and some cited only flulike symptoms or localized reactions at the injection site resulting in discomfort, medical costs, or enforced absence from work. In addition, there were claims alleging that the vaccine had directly caused a wide variety of other problems, including heart attacks, stroke, respiratory disorders, fainting, vision problems, and sexual impotence.

The claims against the government did not come in all at once. The Federal Tort Claims Act includes a statute of limitations that allows a claimant two years after the injury has taken place in which to file his or her claim. Thus, when the Justice Department's lawyer in charge of swine flu litigation, Neil R. Peterson, testified before the Rogers Health Subcommittee oversight hearing on swine flu in September of 1977, he reported that only 743 claims for personal injury had thus far been filed, seeking $325,671,708 in damages. In addition, there were 67 claims of "wrongful death" (including 19 deaths allegedly due to GBS), seeking damages in the amount of $1,032,948,179. This last sum was skewed by a single claim for $1 billion in damages (which was disallowed by the government and subsequently withdrawn). At that point, claims were still being filed at the rate of about twenty per week, and Peterson projected that some 2,500 claims against the government might ultimately be made.[85]

By February 1978, when the final report on the swine flu program was made to Congress, 1241 claims (including 103 for wrongful death) had been filed, seeking over $608 million in damages.[86] As of May 1980, the total number of claims filed was 3,917, for a total of over $3.5 billion in damages. Of these, only 241 have been settled, with the payment of $9.1 million in damages.

The legal process for settling the swine flu claims under the Federal Tort Claims Act was moving more slowly than anyone (except perhaps the lawyers) had expected, and complaints about Justice Department foot-dragging grew more numerous and more vocal. In many parts of the country, the victims of real or imagined vaccine-induced injuries organized committees to press their complaints, and a Guillain-Barré newsletter was started. Complaints about the slowness of the governmental response reached such a pitch that in June of 1978, HEW Secretary Califano announced that the government was desirous of speedily compensating Guillain-Barré Syndrome cases and that it would reduce the burden of proof required of plaintiffs. But follow-up efforts by Justice

Department lawyers to settle these cases administratively proved fruitless. The amount of money that the government felt to be fair compensation was far below what the victims of GBS or their families felt to be equitable, and out-of-court settlement proved impossible in most cases.

The legal process of deciding who had a valid claim against the government because of the aftereffects of immunization, and how much compensation should be awarded, would thus have to be decided by the courts in a slow and arduous process. As of early 1980, only 1,108 claims had been carried to the courts as lawsuits, including 650 GBS cases and 118 wrongful deaths. Many of these have been grouped together for the purposes of trial in federal court, but it will obviously be years before the federal government sees the end of swine flu litigation, and before the full cost of the swine flu program can be fixed with certainty. Whatever the final outcome, the total cost of the program to the American taxpayer will clearly be far less than had earlier been claimed by the insurance industry and by the program's opponents, but far more than had been predicted by the program's supporters.

The tort claims legislation covering the swine flu program had required that HEW explore alternative options for the insurance coverage of future programs and report back to Congress the results of this study. No one wished this ad hoc solution to establish a precedent for all federal public health programs, and Congress worried about the status of even the usual immunization programs other than influenza. Congressman Rogers, who was especially interested in this question, let it be known that his subcommittee expected a comprehensive and useful document. To respond to this charge, Assistant Secretary Cooper appointed an interagency committee within the Public Health Service to explore the possibilities. In addition, he organized two national immunization conferences to examine all aspects of future federal undertakings in this area, in fulfillment of a pledge exacted by Senator Kennedy during a hearing on the polio immunization program in September 1976. One of the topics on the agenda of these conferences was liability, and the report of the liability work group also went to Cooper's interagency committee.[87]

However, the emergency was finally over. During 1977, HEW found that the normal childhood immunization programs were not threatened by liability problems. They could be carried on as usual, as long as the states rather than the federal government assumed the contractual duty to warn vaccine recipients of the risks involved. Neither the manufacturers nor their insurers objected to this procedure, since they felt that the states provided less attractive targets for lawsuit than did the federal government. In addition, the childhood programs were on a far smaller scale and less well advertised than the swine flu effort had been.

In July 1977, long after Cooper had left office, his interagency committee in HEW emerged with a draft report on the liability question, which the higher-ups in HEW found to be unsatisfactory. Califano then appointed a new group to look into the question, and after receiving an extension of the statutory deadline, HEW finally sent a report to the Congress in November 1977. This report, a comprehensive review of the liability problem, assessed the issues and outlined available options.[88] None of the solutions proposed seemed very satisfying, however, especially the simplest and seemingly the most logical: to compensate the victims of future immunization programs by administrative process. This approach would cost the victim his right to litigate his complaints in the courts, and was an unpalatable solution to both Justice Department and civilian lawyers.

Since swine flu had vanished and no new pandemic threat of influenza was visible on the horizon, and because the HEW immunization programs were proceeding as usual, the need to solve the liability problem once and for all no longer seemed so urgent. The HEW report was therefore sent to Congress as an analysis, with no specific recommendations. The issues were extremely complex, and neither Califano nor anyone else was prepared to make the difficult decisions unless forced to do so. Now, four years later, the crucial decisions have still not been made, and the next pandemic emergency threatens to find the country equally unprepared in the critical area of insurance liability.

Fixing the "Blame"

The swine flu program has been labeled a fiasco by Harry Schwartz, and by Secretary Califano, and it was generally perceived as such by the public. In addition to the cost in life and personal injury due to vaccine side effects, and to the still unknown sums that the government would pay to satisfy all valid claims against it, HEW spent directly on the program something over $100 million, and state and local health agencies are estimated to have expended an additional $24 million of their own funds. The CDC purchased over 156 million doses of swine flu vaccine and, worst of all, had over 90 million useless doses of vaccine in storage when the program was terminated.[89] In most such situations, and especially in large organizations like the federal government, the temptation to assign blame is almost irresistible. The notion that things can go so disastrously wrong without someone being at fault is generally difficult to maintain.

One of the first actions taken by incoming Secretary Califano was to notify Assistant Secretary for Health Cooper that he would be replaced, despite Cooper's impressive degree of credibility within both Washington political circles and the health and scientific communities, and despite hints that Cooper would have liked to stay on. It is, of course, the prerogative of a new administration to "clean house" and of a new Cabinet member to bring in his own people. Yet, many observers consider that Cooper was the first and most important casualty of the reaction to the abortive swine flu program.

Next it was Sencer's turn. On February 4, he was called to Washington by Under Secretary of Health, Education, and Welfare, Hale Champion and given notice that he would be replaced as Director of CDC. Sencer asked for and obtained some time to consider his options, and was promised that the news would not be leaked out prematurely. But at the February 7 meeting of the ad hoc committee to consider the moratorium, which was well covered by the press and television, word of Sencer's firing leaked out. On hearing this, Califano called Sencer aside for a private conversation, and that afternoon announced his dismissal on national television at an impromptu press conference. Califano complimented Sencer for his long and distinguished service, but it was clear to everyone that Sencer was the second victim of the swine flu debacle, and many people faulted Califano for the manner and the apparent suddenness of the firing. The CDC people and the scientists present were appalled. It seemed a cruel way to reward an otherwise distinguished career of public service and devotion to one's agency. Morale in the Atlanta agency, already suffering from the immunization program's setbacks, took a nosedive.

Not long after the February 5 decision to lift the moratorium, Secretary Califano commissioned a study of the entire swine flu program. The purpose of the analysis was to review and reconstruct the entire sequence of events, in order to provide lessons for future policy making. He chose for the study Professor Richard E. Neustadt, of the John F. Kennedy School of Government at Harvard, and Dr. Harvey V. Fineberg, Director of the Graduate Program in Health Policy and Management at the Harvard School of Public Health. These authors have provided a comprehensive review of the salient events that contributed to the decisions made concerning swine flu and the implementation of the immunization program.[90] They conclude that seven principal features characterized the program, and contributed to its ultimate failure.

1. Neustadt and Fineberg suggest that the scientists had too much confidence in their theories about the epidemiology of influenza and the biology of the virus, based upon far too meager evidence.

2. They imply that the strong conviction of the scientists, and especially of government health officials, was fueled by a variety of pre-

existing "personal agendas." Time and again the authors hint at seemingly nefarious motives on the part of one or another of the principal actors, and they appear almost unwilling to concede any honorable basis for action to certain of the participants, most notably CDC's Sencer.

3. They suggest that there was an almost unhealthy zeal by the government health professionals to make their lay superiors "do the right thing." Neustadt and Fineberg appear to agree that Sencer, by the words he chose in drafting his action memorandum, "held a gun to the head of the President" and forced Ford to accede to the recommendation for a National Immunization Program.

4. The authors conclude that Sencer and his advisers, with Cooper's acquiescence, made many decisions and commitments prematurely, that is, decided too much too early.

5. They accuse the planners of failing to address the many uncertainties in the program, and of not building in a mechanism for periodic formal reconsideration of the program's direction, or even of its need.

6. They maintain that throughout the course of the program, its logical basis in science was insufficiently questioned as was the prospect for its successful implementation with respect to vaccine production and distribution to the public.

7. They accuse all the government health officials, and the CDC especially, of profound insensitivity in their relations with the news media and in their failure to consider what the program's failure might do to federal health agencies and to their other programs.

Finally, the authors rejected the notion that politics, partisan or otherwise, had any effect on the sequence of events.

It is clear that the Neustadt-Fineberg report represents a severe indictment of government health officials and of most of the outside scientific advisers involved in the swine flu program. The conclusions contained in the report appear to justify the term *fiasco* applied to the program, as well as Califano's firing of Sencer and Cooper as the two main culprits in the piece. In the next chapter, we shall explore in somewhat greater detail whether this analysis was correct, and whether these indictments were justified.

CHAPTER 14

The Lessons of '76

T HE foregoing chapters have attempted to provide enough
detail on the events of 1976, to give the reader a good idea of
what had occurred in connection with swine influenza. It is equally important, however, for the reader to understand *why* things happened as they
did. To this end, a variety of background details in other areas has been
added to the swine flu story. Thus, to understand why the scientific advisers acted as they did in the spring of 1976, it is crucial to examine what
the scientists thought they knew *at that time* about influenza the virus and
influenza the disease. No matter that the future might show their predictions to be wrong; most of today's decisions must be made today and cannot await tomorrow's new facts and insights. Similarly, the actions of
government public health officials cannot be fully understood without
knowing their statutory mission; their own perception of the importance
to their work of such disciplines as preventive medicine; and the structure
of the federal bureaucracy, which imposes a curious relationship between
the full-time, technically trained bureaucrat at the bottom and the transient, politically trained bureaucrat at the top. Finally, the actions of
elected officials, whether in the Congress or the executive branch, cannot
be fully appreciated without some knowledge of the personal styles of the
individuals involved as well as of the contemporary politics of their institutions. It is factors like these that make governmental policy making so
fascinating, and at the same time so frustratingly complex.

Does the "failure" of a major national program like swine flu immunization necessarily imply the existence of a "culprit" responsible for this
failure? The answer to this question must inevitably be yes, if it can be
shown unequivocally that either the initial decision to act was patently
erroneous in terms of the information then available or that the implementation of the program was so inept as to assure failure. The current
popular view, espoused by Harry Schwartz and Joseph Califano and
seemingly confirmed by the Neustadt-Fineberg report, is that the program was indeed a fiasco, and that "too much was decided too early,"
notably by Sencer, Cooper, and their scientific advisers. We will examine

this question in some detail by referring to the swine flu story as recounted in these pages. If the accusations are indeed true, then important changes must be made in our federal health bureaucracy. If the accusations are false, then the record should be corrected, so that the public health establishment will not suffer unwarranted restraints when faced by some future public health emergency.

In order to gain some additional perspective on the swine flu affair of 1976, it might be useful to consider what would have happened had virulent swine flu actually struck in the fall or winter of that year. In the midst of such an epidemic, with millions falling ill all around the country and a rapidly rising "excess mortality," appeals for nonexistent swine flu vaccine and complaints about the inadequacies of the immunization program would have reached a very shrill level indeed. In the stormy aftermath of that type of fiasco, HEW Secretary Califano could well be pictured commissioning an analogous study to find out what had gone wrong, resulting in the probable indictment of Sencer and Cooper for having decided too little too late!

The Initial Decision to Immunize

When swine flu broke out at Fort Dix in early 1976, it seemed almost to write its own scenario, prescribing many of the events that followed. The new virus contained a *double antigenic shift,* hitherto a sure sign of impending pandemic. It appeared at approximately the right time to confirm the *eleven-year cycle* that influenza scientists had predicted as the established pattern for epidemic influenza. Moreover, it was *swine flu with human-to-human transmission,* raising the specter of another deadly 1918–19 catastrophe in a population that had lost its immunity to this strain. This was what the flu experts thought they knew at that time, and it represented the only basis they had for their recommendations. They could not then know what the future would show — that the new strain would confound all of their predictions by disappearing as mysteriously as it had come, rather than spreading through the country and the world in an ever more virulent form.

We have seen that the science of influenza is impure, in the sense that firm predictions cannot be made about its coming and going, nor, even, can educated guesses be made about the probabilities involved in such occurrences. The experts have been criticized for their inability to estimate either the likelihood that pandemic swine flu would return during the following influenza season, or the potential severity of the disease in terms of morbidity and mortality. This criticism is valid, of course, since the experts did not and still do not know how to make such predictions. But the criticism itself may be pointless, inasmuch as it suggests a lack of understanding of the very basis of preventive medicine and of the realities of the real world of politics.

As its name implies, the purpose of preventive medicine is to *prevent* disease. While some programs operate on an individual basis, most preventive medicine approaches seek to *limit the incidence* of disease in entire populations. Examples of this are programs to reduce cholesterol in the diet to prevent heart disease, fluoridation of drinking water to prevent dental caries, or mass immunization campaigns against infectious diseases. Such programs are not considered to be faulty if some proportion of the treated population subsequently develops the disease; it suffices that the preventive medicine program significantly reduces the incidence of disease in the entire population. In this respect, immunization programs against infectious diseases have long proved to be among the most effective forms of preventive medicine.

Just as the presence of some individual illness should not indict a program designed to prevent that illness, failure of the disease to appear at all should not be used to call a program into question. Some preventive medicine programs assume the form of an insurance policy. Few of us condemn ourselves for having paid last year's premium on our home fire insurance policy just because the house did not burn down. Pre-school-age children throughout the United States and much of the world are required by law to be immunized against diphtheria, pertussis (whooping cough), and tetanus (DPT), even though these diseases are rarely seen in this country. This does not mean that the DPT-immunization program is a questionable "waste," any more than that last year's total expenditures by the Department of Defense were a total waste merely because the United States did not suffer military attack. Rather, such programs are designed to reduce the probability of severe attack by some lurking enemy, or to minimize the consequences if the attack does occur. Failure of the attack to come, even if not the direct result of the prevention efforts, should not of itself condemn that program.

The principal criterion for deciding whether or not to embark on a preventive medicine program involves a comparison of the risks (costs) and the potential benefits, to the extent that each can be estimated. The cost of the venture includes not only dollars expended, but some calculation of the likely extent and severity of its harmful side effects. The benefits are measured in terms of the alleviation of suffering and the saving of life, as well as in the economic saving of health care costs, lost productivity, and wages. Such estimates of costs and benefits are usually very difficult to make with any precision, and this was especially true of the swine flu program. In March of 1976, the potential benefits appeared to be the substantial protection of some 60 to 80 percent of the population, the prevention of some tens of thousands of excess deaths, and the possible saving of billions of dollars in economic costs. At that time, the counterbalancing risks were felt to be the $135 million cost of the program, a small proportion of minor ailments due to the flu shot itself, and a very limited number of more serious side effects and even an occasional death. The gamble appeared well worth taking, even if the probability of return of swine flu was small. No one in March could have foreseen Legionnaires' Disease or Guillain-Barré Syndrome, or the tens or hundreds of millions of dollars that would be required to compensate the victims of the latter disease.

Based upon what was known in early 1976, the recommendation of a national immunization program by the scientific advisory panels and by the federal public health officials appeared to represent a reasonable preventive medicine decision.

With substantial unanimity in the scientific community, the political realities enforced acquiescence by those in command in HEW, in the White House, and in the Congress, whose statutory duty it is to make or to agree to the final decision. It mattered little that the experts could not tell whether the chance of pandemic influenza was 30 percent, or 3 percent, or even less than 1 percent. What the assistant secretary for Health, the secretary of HEW, the president, and Congress heard was that there was *some* chance of pandemic flu, and this was enough. No responsible politician at any level wished to put himself in the position of opposing the program, thus running the risk that pandemic illness and death might prove him a villain in the piece. Someone had said early in March, "Suppose there is a pandemic accompanied by death. Then it comes out: they had the opportunity to save life . . . they did nothing." No bureaucrat would wish to face such a charge from his superiors, nor would any politician wish to face it from his electorate.

The alternative was a national program that would cost *only* $135 million. While this seems like a lot of money to the average citizen, it is not a large sum to those in the executive or legislative branches used to dealing with billions of dollars. It calls to mind Everett Dirksen's wry remark that "a billion dollars here, and a billion dollars there, and pretty soon you're talking about *real* money!" With a national budget measured in the hundreds of billions of dollars, $135 million seemed like only a modest sum to gamble on the politically sensitive issue of the health of the American people.

The charge has been made that the scientists, with their recommendation for a national influenza program, and Sencer, with his action memorandum, "held a gun to the head of the President" and *forced* him to go along with the program. In the broadest sense, the accusation is true, but it seems somehow misplaced. Certainly it was the event itself — the outbreak of swine flu at Fort Dix — that forced the issue on everyone involved: scientists, bureaucrats, the president, and Congress. We must be careful to resist the temptation to punish the messenger who brings the bad news.

The swine flu affair brings into sharp focus the curious relationship that exists between scientific advisers and the government they serve. The layman (and the politician) somehow persist in their belief that Science deals in absolute and immutable truths, and consequently they are repeatedly frustrated when scientists testify on all sides of important national issues like energy, the safety of nuclear plants, safeguarding the environment, or the integrity of the ozone layer above the earth. When the public and the politician expect clear pronouncements from a scientific monolith, they often find reputable scientists differing not only on the solutions to problems but even on whether the problems exist. Does saccharine cause cancer? Can we and should we spend $10 to $20 billion to put a man on the moon? Should we concentrate our present efforts on solar energy, or on nuclear fusion, to solve the energy problem? "Science" cannot provide definitive answers to most of these questions; at best, it can only provide the best information it has at the time, even if it is uncertain and conflicting. In our society, it is ultimately the politician who must decide on these matters, and woe betide the politician who neglects political realities: the perceived needs of the society, the concerns and clamor of his constituents, the economic and political costs of the various solutions, and the relative value of other desirable programs within the limitations of a finite budget.

When, however, a national "emergency" arises which finds the scientific community in substantial unanimity on a course of action (and especially in the area of health), then it is doubly difficult for the lay politician to resist. Where else could he turn for advice on an issue like swine flu in 1976? Should the HEW secretary have formed an independent scientific panel competent to pass judgment on the validity of the recommendations made by Sencer and his advisory committee? Should Ford have been able to refer the question to a presidential Office of Science and Technology Planning? Should Congress have had the in-house scientific competence to weigh the recommendation? Ideally, the answer to each must be yes, but practically such multiple layers of scientific review would be meaningless. The number of world-renowned influenza scientists can almost be counted on the fingers of both hands, and most of these participated in one way or another in the initial decision. Anyone, even another scientist seeking to advise the secretary, the president, or Congress, would have to consult among this small group, and this in fact was done by Sencer, by Cooper, by those who advised Mathews, Ford, and the Congress, and at the White House meeting itself.

The pejorative charge is made that scientific subspecialities such as influenza virology are ruled by closed cliques that are inbred and self-serving. This charge is basically true, but it is difficult to see how it might be otherwise. The few leading specialists in any scientific field meet continually with one another to discuss their common interests and the latest data. They are invited to the same advisory committees and scientific symposia, and they train the next generation of scientists in their laboratories. If this puts the policy-making generalist in a position of great dependence upon the competence of the scientists and technicians under him, then so be it. Whether in government or industry, the final decision is his. That is what he is elected or hired to do, as explicitly stated in his contract with his constituents or with his board of directors.

The same type of argument applies to the charge that the swine flu decision was made without adequate input from the public. While "the public" certainly has a right to know about governmental decisions in the making, on what basis can it intelligently participate in the day-to-day operations of government? Where is it to get *its* expertise? On any public question such as swine flu, there will always be a Harry Schwartz to question whether government should properly engage in such public health ventures, a Ralph Nader to claim that swine flu will not return and that the program is a waste, or a J. Anthony Morris to claim that the flu vaccine is not only ineffective but actually harmful. These voices were heard, however, in the pages of the *New York Times,* at congressional hearings, and on national television. While informed public participation on such matters should be encouraged in our society — if often more for form than for substance — it is arguable whether the swine flu outcome in 1976 would have been changed by "opening up" the process further. Indeed, Secretary Califano did just this, opening his ad hoc immunization meetings to broad public participation and to the news media, yet the recommendations that emerged were precisely those required by the circumstances at that time. Ultimately, the public does express its approval or disapproval. It votes with its feet, in deciding whether to line up for the vaccine, and with its ballots, in assessing how well its representatives have served it.

The initial decision on swine flu was really a double one: first, whether to act and produce vaccine, and second, whether to schedule the immunizations or hold off and stockpile the vaccine. Once again, it was a question of whether or not to believe the experts who claimed that once the pandemic arrived there would not be time to get the vaccine out of storage and into people's arms. Their recommendation was based upon three factors: (1) the unhappy experiences of 1957 and 1968, when vaccine distribution was so unsatisfactory; (2) the knowledge that if the pandemic came, they would be indicted by an angry public demanding to know why the protective vaccine was sitting in cold storage; and (3) their belief that the vaccine was safe. We may never know whether the experts were correct in rejecting the stockpile option. Or perhaps we may find out after all, when the next influenza pandemic strikes.

Implementation of the Immunization Program

A review of the events from March to December of 1976 suggests that those responsible for the implementation of the National Influenza Immunization Program were guilty of extreme overoptimism at best and of unfortunate naiveté at worst. In order to achieve the goals originally set by the Advisory Committee on Immunization Practices and by the CDC, and declared in somewhat expanded form by President Ford, *everything* had to work perfectly and with clockwork precision. The manufacturers had to start production immediately and maintain an uninterrupted maximum effort throughout the program. Two doses of vaccine had to be harvested from each infected egg; and the technical processes involved in virus purification, inactivation, the preparation of split virus, and subsequent safety testing had to proceed without a hitch. It was necessary that a single dose of vaccine produce adequate immunity in substantially all of the population, including children. It was critical for the program that all levels of both public and private health sectors not only be imbued with a positive attitude toward the program but also be efficiently mobilized in order to achieve maximum distribution of the vaccine when it became available. Finally, and perhaps most importantly, the general public had to be made to feel that the program was warranted and the vaccine desirable. In the end, *not one* of the aspects of the program worked out quite the way it had originally been envisaged.

As we learned from the preceding pages, almost everything that *could* have gone wrong with the program *did* go wrong; but as we also learned, few of the problems could have been precisely predicted beforehand. This fact, however, does not exculpate the program's managers. It only serves to point out the inherent defect of planning a program based upon optimistic "best-case" rather than upon pessimistic "worst-case" estimates. What is probably required in such ventures is an approach that involves hoping for the best, but preparing for the worst.

From the earliest stages of the program, and throughout its existence, the planners would have benefited immeasurably by having a group of knowledgeable and practical people to do little other than to explore the possible workings of Murphy's law on the swine flu program. *What if* the yield per egg is less than two doses of vaccine? *What if* the field trials show that a single dose of vaccine is less effective than predicted, or that children with little immunologic "knowledge" of flu viruses do not respond to the vaccine with adequate immunity, or *what if* vaccine side effects prove to be more severe than expected? *What if* the improbable occurs, and a few people drop dead of heart attacks in the immunization lines? *What if* swine flu comes prematurely, before the populace has been immunized? *What more should we do* to assure the cooperation and organization of those who will administer the vaccine? *What more should we do* to help the mass media educate the public, and to help defuse negative influences on the program? And, finally, questions should continually have been asked in the form, *What are the implications for the program* of . . .? In April and May of 1976, someone knowledgeable should have asked what were the implications for the program of the increasing rumblings about insurance liability emanating from the vaccine manufacturers and later from the insurance industry. In June, the same questions should have been seriously asked about children's shots, and about the defection of Drs. Sabin and Alexander to the ranks of those who advocated stockpiling the vaccine and holding off on the immunization program. In August, someone should have examined the implications of the serious production lags that had resulted from the delayed settlement of the insurance liability controversy.

Who should have asked these questions? The scientists and public health experts who possess the expertise required to make the original recommendations generally do not have practical experience in the world of large-scale production and distribution, or in the complexities of accounting and legal practices. They tend rather to be eternal optimists, more accustomed to and comfortable with theory than practice. Even the specialists at CDC and BoB, experienced in far more modest programs on a nonemergency basis, were at a disadvantage in dealing with the swine flu program in terms of its size, scope, crisis deadlines, and unprecedented high-level sponsorship. What was sorely needed here was a small group of individuals trained in the practical problems of production and distribution, and who knew from experience how vindictive Murphy's law can really be. Needed by the program, but unavailable in 1976, were production experts from industry, logistics experts, lawyers, public relations people, and even politicians. Such individuals could have assisted the public health professionals immeasurably, by questioning the assumptions upon which policy decisions were based, the optimistic forecasts of accomplishments, and the validity of goals. Most important, such a group could have more than paid its way simply by brainstorming Murphy's law, and exploring what it could do to the National Immunization Program. Nelson Rockefeller may have been correct in thinking that logistics experts in the armed services might do a better job than those in HEW.

The Next Great Plague

Despite the failure of swine flu to return as predicted in 1976, everything that we know about the molecular biology of the flu virus and about the epidemiology of influenza suggests that, *sooner or later,* severe pandemic influenza will once again ravage the world. What will happen when it returns? Of course, if it appears somewhere in Asia during the summer months, and immediately spreads around the world exacting its toll in illness and death, then little will be done owing to lack of time. But suppose that it crops up somewhere in February or March, giving enough warning to permit the public health establishment to prepare to deal with it. Will the politicians and the public respond to an appeal for an immunization program, or will they turn a deaf ear, concluding that the experts had cried "wolf" once too often in 1976?

It may even be fair to ask whether scientific advisers and federal health officials will even dare to ask for such a program the next time, since they seem to have been so badly burned by the events of 1976. Will a future Director of CDC or a future assistant secretary of health be brave enough to advise another National Immunization Program, having seen the previous one labeled a fiasco and resulting in the dismissal of the CDC director and the assistant secretary who recommended it? Or will the experts and the politicians wait until the pandemic is upon us and the morbidity and the mortality figures are rising before daring to act? One hopes that by then, the swine flu affair of 1976 will be seen in a more reasonable perspective, and that further research on the elusive flu virus will allow more dependable predictions to be made.

The Lessons

The story told in the previous chapters suggests the following conclusions:

1. *The decision in March of 1976 to mount a National Immunization Program against swine flu was correct.* Everything that was known about the science of influenza at that time suggested that the pandemic might come

and that there was time to help protect the public from its ravages. While certain actions may have been colored by the possibility of personal, scientific, institutional, or political gain, we must conclude that all of the participants, including Sencer, Cooper, Mathews, Ford, and the scientific advisers acted in what they felt were the best interests of the American people.

2. *The initial decision to vaccinate the public rather than stockpile the vaccine was correct.* Given the possibility of a pandemic, the rapidity of spread of influenza, and the previous safety record of influenza vaccines, this decision appeared reasonable in March. This is not to say, however, that the decision could not and should not have been reconsidered in August, when swine flu had failed to appear in the Southern Hemisphere during its flu season, when production schedules were falling far behind due to the insurance controversy, and when public acceptance of the program had started to wane.

3. *The National Immunization Program was administered conscientiously, if somewhat ineptly, by those in charge.* The program managers do not appear to be guilty of any serious errors of commission. Rather, they may be accused of overoptimism and of failing to anticipate or prepare adequately for inevitable problems, such as the Pittsburgh deaths and the education of the nation's health establishment, the news media, and the public.

4. *There were no real "culprits" in 1976.* Everyone involved with the swine flu affair seems to have been conscientiously attempting to do his best, but all were caught up in a vortex of unpredictable events. The scientists suffered from the lack of precision that accompanies any impure science, while the governmental program managers suffered from their lack of experience in ventures of this type and magnitude. All were at the mercy of unpredictable events. If there were any culprits, then it was swine flu, which failed to appear and "justify" the program of preventive medicine; or it was Legionnaires' Disease, which in August resurrected the program that perhaps should have been allowed to expire quietly at that point; and most certainly, it was the unpredictable Guillain-Barré Syndrome, which forced the program's demise and assured it the persisting label of fiasco.

There are, however, lessons to be learned and benefits to be derived even from program failures. This is especially true of the swine flu affair, since pandemic influenza will surely return sometime in the future when an appropriate antigenic shift takes place again, and must somehow be coped with. Future timidity, based upon a misunderstanding of what occurred in 1976, may make us unwilling to take the new gamble on perhaps millions of cases of illness and perhaps tens of thousands of deaths. We would hope, however, that the federal government will acknowledge its unique responsibilities in this area, and act. But things should be done somewhat differently the next time, based upon what we have already learned. Among the lessons for the next time are:

1. The decision to produce vaccine should probably be separated from the decision to immunize. Each action should have its own well-defined triggers, such as the appearance of a specified number of outbreaks of a specified severity in certain geographic locations.

2. The final announcement to act and commitment of prestige of person or of office should be made at the lowest level of bureaucracy practicable, rather than at the highest. Perhaps Gerald Ford was right in 1976 in thinking that only the prestige of the presidency could assure successful implementation of the swine flu immunization program. But in doing so, he severely limited the options of those below him in HEW to reconsider, and of those in Congress to question.

3. A mechanism should be built into such programs from the start which requires periodic reevaluation of the premises upon which decisions are made and reconsideration of those decisions based upon the latest available information. What appears imperative in February or March may no longer seem justified in August or September.

4. All predictions and timetables must be questioned and requestioned. Some specialists (preferably outsiders) must be assigned to think about the possible effects of Murphy's law.

5. The professionals who recommend a future program should not be left to manage it alone. They will most likely need the help of individuals with more practical experience in management, in production, in logistics, in law, and in other fields.

6. Closer attention must be paid to public relations. Better mechanisms must be established to reach and adequately inform the public and private health communities and the general public itself. Those in the health sector must gain a better understanding of how the news media function, and attempt to educate the media about how they function.

7. The insurance liability problem must be solved in advance. It is a serious problem, one that is still with us and still extremely complicated. We cannot again afford to devote another two or three months to putting together a new ad hoc and perhaps unsatisfying solution, while the program languishes.

If we are willing to learn from our past mistakes, then the "next time" may prove a happier experience than did the swine flu affair of 1976.

APPENDIX A / Sencer's Action Memorandum

MEMORANDUM

DEPARTMENT OF HEALTH, EDUCATION, AND WELFARE
OFFICE OF THE ASSISTANT SECRETARY FOR HEALTH

TO : The Secretary
Through: ES *DHK*/*K*

DATE: **MAR 1 8 1976**

FROM : Assistant Secretary for Health

SUBJECT: Swine Influenza--ACTION

ISSUE

How should the Federal Government respond to the influenza problem
caused by a new virus?

FACTS

1. In February 1976 a new strain of influenza virus, designated as
influenza A/New Jersey/76 (Hsw1N1), was isolated from an outbreak of
disease among recruits in training at Fort Dix, New Jersey.

2. The virus is antigenically related to the influenza virus which
has been implicated as the cause of the 1918-1919 pandemic which
killed 450,000 people--more than 400 of every 100,000 Americans.

3. The entire U.S. population under the age of 50 is probably
susceptible to this new strain.

4. Prior to 1930, this strain was the predominate cause of human
influenza in the U.S. Since 1930, the virus has been limited to
transmission among swine with only occasional transmission from swine
to man--with no secondary person-to-person transmission.

5. In an average year, influenza causes about 17,000 deaths (9 per
100,000 population) and costs the nation approximately $500 million.

6. Severe epidemics, or pandemics, of influenza occur at approximately
10 year intervals. In 1968-69, influenza struck 20 percent of our population,
causing more than 33,000 deaths (14 per 100,000) and cost an estimated
$3.2 billion.

7. A vaccine to protect against swine influenza can be developed before
the next flu season; however, the production of large quantities would
require extraordinary efforts by drug manufacturers.

The Secretary   2

ASSUMPTIONS

1. Although there has been only one outbreak of A/swine influenza,
person-to-person spread has been proven and additional outbreaks
cannot be ruled out. Present evidence and past experience indicate
a strong possibility that this country will experience widespread
A/swine influenza in 1976-77. Swine flu represents a major antigenic
shift from recent viruses and the population under 50 is almost universally
susceptible. These are the ingredients for a pandemic.

2. Routine public health influenza recommendations (immunization of the
population at high risk--elderly and chronically ill persons) would
not forestall a flu pandemic. Routine actions would have to be
supplemented.

3. The situation is one of "go or no go". If extraordinary measures
are to be undertaken there is barely enough time to assure adequate
vaccine production and to mobilize the nation's health care delivery
system. Any extensive immunization program would have to be in full
scale operation by the beginning of September and should not last beyond
the end of November 1976. A decision must be made now.

4. There is no medical epidemiologic basis for excluding any part of the
population--swine flu vaccine will be recommended for the total population
except in individual cases. Similarly there is no public health or
epidemiologic rationale for narrowing down the targeted population.
Further, it is assumed that it would be socially and politically unacceptable
to plan for less than 100 percent coverage. Therefore, it is assumed that
any recommendations for action must be directed toward the goal of
immunizing 213 million people in three months (September through November
1976). The nation has never attempted an immunization program of such
scope and intensity.

5. A public health undertaking of this magnitude cannot succeed without
Federal leadership, sponsorship, and some level of financial support.

6. The vaccine when purchased in large quantities will cost around
50 cents per dose. Nationally, the vaccine will cost in excess of
$100 million. To this total must be added delivery costs, as well as
costs related to surveillance and monitoring. Part, but not all, of the
costs can be considered sunk costs, or as non-additive. Regardless of
what strategy is adopted, it will be extremely difficult to estimate
the amount of additional costs that will result from a crash influenza
immunization program.

The Secretary   3

7. The Advisory Committee on Immunization Practices will recommend
formally and publicly, the immunization of the total U.S. population
against A/swine influenza.

8. Any recommended course of action, other than no action, must assure:

--that a supply of vaccine is produced which is adequate to immunize
the whole population.

--that adequate supplies of vaccine are available as needed at health
care delivery points.

--that the American people are made aware of the need for immunization
against this flu virus.

--that the population systematically reach or be reached by the
health system.

--that the Public Health Service maintain epidemiologic, laboratory,
and immunization surveillance of the population for complications
of vaccination, for influenza morbidity and mortality, and for
vaccine effectiveness and efficacy.

--that the unique research opportunities be maximized.

--that evaluation of the effectiveness of the efforts is conducted.

ALTERNATIVE COURSES OF ACTION

1. No Action

An argument can be made for taking no extraordinary action beyond what
would normally be recommended. To date there has been only one outbreak.
The swine flu virus has been around, but has not caused a problem among
humans since 1930.

Pro:

--The market place would prevail--private industry (drug manufacturers)
would produce in accordance with its estimate of demand and the
consumers would make their own decisions. Similarly, States would
respond in accordance with their own sets of priorities.

--The "pandemic" might not occur and the Department would have
avoided unnecessary health expenditures.

--Any real action would require direct Federal intervention which is
contrary to current administration philosophy.

The Secretary   4

Con:

--Congress, the media, and the American people will expect some action.

--The Administration can tolerate unnecessary health expenditures better than unnecessary death and illness, particularly if a flu pandemic should occur.

--In all likelihood, Congress will act on its own initiative.

2. Minimum Response

Under this option there would be a limited Federal role with primary reliance on delivery systems now in place and on spontaneous, non-governmental action.

   a. The Federal Government would advise the drug industry to develop and produce A/swine vaccine sufficient to immunize the general population. The Federal Government would underwrite this effort by promising to purchase vaccine for the 58 million Federal beneficiaries.

   b. A nationwide public awareness program would be undertaken to serve as general backdrop for local programs.

   c. The Public Health Service would stimulate community programs sponsored by local organizations (medical societies, associations, industries, etc.)

   d. The Center for Disease Control would maintain epidemiologic and laboratory surveillance of the population.

   e. The National Institutes of Health would conduct studies and investigations, particularly on new and improved vaccines.

Pro:

--The approach is characterized by high visability, minimum Federal intervention, and diffused liability and responsibility. It is a partnership with the private sector that relies on Federal stimulation of nongovernmental action.

--The burden on the Federal budget would be minimal. Assuming purchase of vaccines for 58 million beneficiaries, plus additional costs related to c., d., and e., above the total new obligational authority requirement would not exceed $40 million ($32 million for vaccine; plus 8 million for surveillance, monitoring, evaluation, and research).

The Secretary   5

    --Success would depend upon widespread voluntary action--in terms of
    individual choice to seek immunization and in terms of voluntary
    community programs not unlike the polio programs of the past.

    Con:

    --There is little assurance that vaccine manufacturers will undertake
    the massive production effort that would be required to assure
    availability of vaccine for the entire nation.

    --There would be no control over the distribution of vaccines to the
    extent that they are available; the poor, the near poor, and the
    aging usually get left out. Even under routine flu recommendations
    in which the elderly are a primary target, only about half the
    high risk population gets immunized against flu.

    --Probably only about half the population would get immunized.

3. Government Program

This alternative is based on virtually total government responsibility
for the nationwide immunization program.

    a. The Federal Government would advise vaccine manufacturers to
        embark on full scale production of vaccine with the expectation
        of Federal purchase of up to 200 million doses.

    b. The Public Health Service, through the CDC would purchase the
        vaccines for distribution to State Health Departments.

    c. In each State the health department would organize and carry out
        an immunization program designed to reach 100 percent of the State's
        population. Vaccine would be available only through programs
        carried out under the aegis of the State health department
        (or the Federal Government for direct Federal beneficiaries).

    d. Primary reliance would be placed on systematic, planned delivery
        of vaccine in such a way as to make maximum use of intensive,
        high volume immunization techniques and procedures--particularly
        the use of jet-injector guns.

    e. In addition to a general nationwide awareness program, intensive
        promotion and outreach activities would be carried out at the
        local level. Maximum use would be made of temporary employment
        of unemployed workers, high school and college students,
        housewives, and retired people as outreach workers and for jobs
        requiring no special health skills.

The Secretary   6

    f. The Center for Disease Control would maintain epidemiologic and
        laboratory surveillance of the population.

    g. The National Institutes of Health would conduct studies and
        investigations, particularly on new and improved vaccines.

    h. The program would be evaluated to assess the effectiveness of the
        effort in reducing influenza associated morbidity, hospitalization,
        and mortality in a pandemic period.

Pro:

--Under this alternative adequate availability of vaccine would be
  closest to certainty, and the vaccine would be distributed throughout
  the nation most equitably.

--There would be greater certainty of participation of all States
  as well as a predictably more uniform level of intensity across the
  nation.

--Accessibility to immunization services would not depend upon
  economic status.

--This approach would provide the framework for better planning -
  for example, the use of travelling immunization teams which could
  take the vaccine to the people; and greater use of the jet injector,
  and other mass immunization techniques.

--The Federal and State governments traditionally have been responsible
  for the control of communicable diseases; therefore, the strategy
  relies upon government action in an area of public health where the
  States are strong and where basic operating mechanisms exist.

Con:

--This alternative would be very costly and given the timing, the
  magnitude of the problem, and the status of State fiscal health,
  the costs would have to be borne by the Federal Government. The
  impact on the Federal budget would be an increase of $190 million
  in new obligational authority.

--The approach is inefficient to the extent that it fails to take
  advantage of the private sector health delivery system, placing
  too much reliance on public clinics and government action.

The Secretary   7

   --While this approach would undoubtedly result in a higher percentage
   of the population being immunized than would be the case with the
   Minimum Response strategy (alternative 2), it is unlikely that the
   public sector could achieve uniform high levels of protection.
   Although socioeconomic barriers to immunization services would
   be virtually eliminated, breakdowns would occur because the program
   is beyond the scope of official agencies.

   --A totally "public" program is contrary to the spirit and custom
   of health care delivery in this country and should only be
   considered if it is clearly the most effective approach.

4. Combined Approach

A program based on this strategy would take advantage of the strengths
and resources of both the public and private sectors. Successful
immunization of our population in three months' time can be accomplished
only in this manner in this country. In essence, the plan would rely on:
the Federal Government for its technical leadership and coordination,
and its purchase power; State health agencies for their experience in
conducting immunization programs and as logical distribution centers
for vaccine; and on the private sector for its medical and other resources
which must be mobilized.

   a. The Federal Government would advise vaccine manufacturers to
      embark on full scale production of enough vaccine to immunize
      the American people. The Public Health Service would contract
      for 200 million doses of vaccine which would be made available
      at no cost through State health agencies.

   b. State health agencies would develop plans to immunize the people
      in their States through a combination of official and voluntary
      action - travelling immunization teams, community programs,
      private physician practices, as examples.

   c. The strategy would be to tailor the approach to the situation or
      opportunity--using mass immunization techniques where appropriate,
      but also using delivery points already in place such as:
      physicians' offices, health department clinics, community health
      centers--any place with the competence to perform immunization
      services.

   d. Awareness campaigns would be carried out at the local level against
      a broader, generalized nationwide effort. Use would be made of
      unemployed workers, students, etc., for certain jobs.

   e. The Center for Disease Control would maintain epidemiologic and
      laboratory surveillance of the population.

The Secretary   8

    f. The National Institutes of Health would conduct studies and
        investigations of vaccine effectiveness and efficacy.

    g. The program would be evaluated to assess the effectiveness of the
        effort in reducing influenza associated morbidity, hospitalization,
        and mortality in a pandemic period.

Pro:

--Under this alternative adequate availability of vaccine would be
  closest to certainty, and the vaccine would be distributed throughout
  the nation most equitably.

--There would be greater certainty of participation of all States
  as well as a predictably more uniform level of intensity across
  the nation.

--Accessibility to immunization services would not depend upon
  socioeconomic factors.

--Making use of all delivery points better assures that the vaccine
  will get to more people.

--The approach provides the framework for planning and expands the
  scope of resources which can be applied.

--Undertaking the program in this manner provides a practical,
  contemporary example of government, industry, and private citizens
  cooperating to serve a common cause.

Con:

--This strategy would require substantial Federal expenditures. A
  supplemental request of approximately $134 million would be needed.

--Under this alternative there is the greatest possibility of some
  people being needlessly reimmunized.

DISCUSSION

Any of the courses of action would raise budgetary and authorization
questions and these will be discussed later. More important is the question
of what the Federal Government is willing to invest if some action is
deemed necessary to avert a possible influenza pandemic. We have not
undertaken a health program of this scope and intensity before in our
history. There are no precedents, nor mechanisms in place that are suited

The Secretary   9

to an endeavor of this magnitude. Given this situation, can we afford
the administrative and programmatic inflexibility that would result from
normal considerations about duplicative costs, third party reimbursements,
and Federal-State or public-private relationships and responsibilities?
The magnitude of the challenge suggests that the Department must either
be willing to take extraordinary steps or be willing to accept an approach
to the problem that cannot succeed.

It is recommended that the Department, through the Public Health Service
and the Center for Disease Control, undertake an influenza immunization
campaign as outlined in alternative 4, <u>Combined Approach</u>. This alternative
best satisfies all of the minimum program requirements outlined earlier
and more importantly, it is the most likely to succeed--more people would
be protected.

The question of legislative authorization is not entirely clear. It
would appear that Section 311 a. of the Public Health Service Act contains
adequate authority to implement the recommended program. If 311 a. cannot
be used, then it will be necessary to seek "point of order" authority
in the supplemental appropriation act. It is anticipated that Congress
would be receptive to "point of order" language in this instance.

It will be necessary to seek a supplemental appropriation so that all
parties can begin to mobilize for the big push in the fall. It will also
be necessary for the funds to be available until expended because the
program, although time-limited, falls into fiscal year 1976, the transition
quarter, and fiscal year 1977. In general terms the request would be for
approximately $134 million made up as follows:

    Immunization Programs
      (vaccines, supplies, temporary personnel,
        awareness) $126 million

    Surveillance and Research   8 million

<u>RECOMMENDATION</u>

It is recommended that the Secretary adopt alternative 4 as the Department's
strategy and that the Public Health Service be given responsibility for
the program and be directed to begin immediate implementation.

                                      James F. Dickson
                           Theodore Cooper, M.D.

APPENDIX B / Public Law 94-266 (Emergency Supplemental Appropriations)

Public Law 94-266
94th Congress, H. J. Res. 890
April 15, 1976

Joint Resolution

Making emergency supplemental appropriations for public employment programs, summer youth programs, and preventive health services for the fiscal year ending June 30, 1976, and for other purposes

Resolved by the Senate and House of Representatives of the United States of America in Congress assembled, That the following sums are appropriated, out of any money in the Treasury not otherwise appropriated, for the fiscal year ending June 30, 1976, namely:

Emergency supplemental appropriations, 1976.

TITLE I

INDEPENDENT AGENCIES

ENVIRONMENTAL PROTECTION AGENCY

CONSTRUCTION GRANTS

For an additional amount for liquidation of obligations incurred pursuant to authority contained in section 203 of the Federal Water Pollution Control Act, as amended, $300,000,000, to remain available until expended.

33 USC 1283.

TITLE II

DEPARTMENT OF LABOR

EMPLOYMENT AND TRAINING ADMINISTRATION

COMPREHENSIVE MANPOWER ASSISTANCE

For an additional amount for "Comprehensive manpower assistance", $528,420,000, to remain available until September 30, 1976.

TEMPORARY EMPLOYMENT ASSISTANCE

For expenses necessary to carry out activities authorized by title II of the Comprehensive Employment and Training Act of 1973, as amended (29 U.S.C. 841–851), $1,200,000,000, to remain available until January 31, 1977.

COMMUNITY SERVICE EMPLOYMENT FOR OLDER AMERICANS

To carry out title IX of the Older Americans Act, as amended, $55,900,000, to remain available until June 30, 1977.

42 USC 3056.

90 STAT. 362

Pub. Law 94-266   - 2 -   April 15, 1976

DEPARTMENT OF HEALTH, EDUCATION, AND WELFARE

CENTER FOR DISEASE CONTROL

PREVENTIVE HEALTH SERVICES

42 USC 241, 289a.

For an additional amount for "Preventive Health Services" for carrying out, to the extent not otherwise provided, title III and section 431 of the Public Health Service Act for a comprehensive, nationwide influenza immunization program, $135,064,000, to remain available until expended: *Provided*, That vaccines may be supplied to State and local health agencies without charge.

RELATED AGENCY

COMMUNITY SERVICES ADMINISTRATION

COMMUNITY SERVICES PROGRAM

For an additional amount for "Community services program", $23,000,000, to remain available until September 30, 1976.

Approved April 15, 1976.

LEGISLATIVE HISTORY:

HOUSE REPORT No. 94-1004 (Comm. on Appropriations).
SENATE REPORT No. 94-742 (Comm. on Appropriations).
CONGRESSIONAL RECORD, Vol. 122 (1976):
    Apr. 5, considered and passed House.
    Apr. 9, considered and passed Senate, amended.
    Apr. 12, House concurred in Senate amendments.
WEEKLY COMPILATION OF PRESIDENTIAL DOCUMENTS, Vol. 12, No. 16:
    Apr. 15, Presidential statement.

90 STAT. 363

APPENDIX C / Public Law 94-380 (National Swine Flu Immunization Program of 1976)

Public Law 94-380
94th Congress, S. 3735
August 12, 1976

An Act

To amend the Public Health Service Act to authorize the establishment and implementation of an emergency national swine flu immunization program and to provide an exclusive remedy for personal injury or death arising out of the manufacture, distribution, or administration of the swine flu vaccine under such program.

Be it enacted by the Senate and House of Representatives of the United States of America in Congress assembled, That this Act may be cited as the "National Swine Flu Immunization Program of 1976".

SEC. 2. Section 317 of the Public Health Service Act (42 U.S.C. 247b) is amended by inserting after subsection (i) the following new subsections:

National Swine Flu Immunization Program of 1976. 42 USC 201 note.

"(j)(1) The Secretary is authorized to establish, conduct, and support (by grant or contract) needed activities to carry out a national swine flu immunization program until August 1, 1977 (hereinafter in this section referred to as the 'swine flu program'). The swine flu program shall be limited to the following:

"(A) The development of a safe and effective swine flu vaccine.

"(B) The preparation and procurement of such vaccine in sufficient quantities for the immunization of the population of the States.

"(C) The making of grants to State health authorities to assist in meeting their costs in conducting or supporting, or both, programs to administer such vaccine to their populations, and the furnishing to State health authorities of sufficient quantities of such swine flu vaccine for such programs.

Grants.

"(D) The furnishing to Federal health authorities of appropriate quantities of such vaccine.

"(E) The conduct and support of training of personnel for immunization activities described in subparagraphs (C) and (D) of this paragraph and the conduct and support of research on the nature, cause, and effect of the influenza against which the swine flu vaccine is designed to immunize, the nature and effect of such vaccine, immunization against and treatment of such influenza, and the cost and effectiveness of immunization programs against such influenza.

"(F) The development, in consultation with the National Commission for the Protection of Human Subjects of Biomedical and Behavioral Research, and implementation of a written informed consent form and procedures for assuring that the risks and benefits from the swine flu vaccine are fully explained to each individual to whom such vaccine is to be administered. Such consultation shall be completed within two weeks after enactment of this Act, or by September 1, 1976, whichever is sooner. Such procedures shall include the information necessary to advice individuals with respect to their rights and remedies arising out of the administration of such vaccine.

Informed consent form and procedures.

"(G) Such other activities as are necessary to implement the swine flu program.

Pub. Law 94-380   - 2 -   August 12, 1976

Reports to
Congress.

"(2) The Secretary shall submit quarterly reports to the Congress on the administration of the swine flu program. Each such report shall provide information on—
"(A) the current supply of the swine flu vaccine to be used in the program;
"(B) the number of persons inoculated with such vaccine since the last report was made under this paragraph and the immune status of the population;
"(C) the amount of funds expended for the swine flu program by the United States, each State, and any other entity participating in the program and the costs of each such participant which are associated with the program, during the period with respect to which the report is made; and
"(D) the epidemiology of influenza in the United States during such period.

Contracts.

"(3) Any contract for procurement by the United States of swine flu vaccine from a manufacturer of such vaccine shall (notwithstanding any other provision of law) be subject to renegotiation to eliminate any profit realized from such procurement (except that with respect to vaccine against the strain of influenza virus known as influenza A/Victoria/75 profit shall be allowed but limited to an amount not exceeding a reasonable profit), as determined pursuant to criteria prescribed by the Secretary, and the contract shall expressly so provide. Such criteria shall specify that any insurance premium amount which is included in the price of such procurement contract and which is refunded to the manufacturer under any retrospective, experience-rating plan or similar rating plan shall in turn be refunded to the United States.

Insurance pre-
mium amounts,
refund.

"(4) No funds are authorized to be appropriated to carry out the activities of the swine flu program authorized in subparagraphs (A), (B), (D), (E), and (F) of paragraph (1) of this subsection in addition to the funds appropriated by Public Law 94-266.

Ante, p. 362.
Claims
against the
United States.

"(k)(1)(A) The Congress finds that—
"(i) in order to achieve the participation in the program of the agencies, organizations, and individuals who will manufacture, distribute, and administer the swine flu vaccine purchased and used in the swine flu program and to assure the availability of such vaccine in interstate commerce, it is necessary to protect such agencies, organizations, and individuals against liability for other than their own negligence to persons alleging personal injury or death arising out of the administration of such vaccine;
"(ii) to provide such protection and to establish an orderly procedure for the prompt and equitable handling of claims by persons alleging such injury or death, it is necessary that an exclusive remedy for such claimants be provided against the United States because of its unique role in the initiation, planning, and administration of the swine flu program; and
"(iii) in order to be prepared to meet the potential emergency of a swine flu epidemic, it is necessary that a procedure be instituted for the handling of claims by persons alleging such injury or death until Congress develops a permanent approach for handling claims arising under programs of the Public Health Service Act.

42 USC 201
note.

August 12, 1976   - 3 -   Pub. Law 94-380

"(B) To—

"(i) assure an orderly procedure for the prompt and equitable handling of any claim for personal injury or death arising out of the administration of such vaccine; and

"(ii) achieve the participation in the swine flu program of (I) the manufacturers and distributors of the swine flu vaccine, (II) public and private agencies or organizations that provide inoculations without charge for such vaccine or its administration and in compliance with the informed consent form and procedures requirements prescribed pursuant to subparagraph (F) of paragraph (1) of this subsection, and (III) medical and other health personnel who provide or assist in providing inoculations without charge for such vaccine or its administration and in compliance with such informed consent form and procedures requirements, it is the purpose of this subsection to establish a procedure under which all such claims will be asserted directly against the United States under section 1346(b) of title 28, United States Code, and chapter 171 of such title (relating to tort claims procedure) except as otherwise specifically provided in this subsection.   28 USC 2671 et seq. Liability.

"(2)(A) The United States shall be liable with respect to claims submitted after September 30, 1976 for personal injury or death arising out of the administration of swine flu vaccine under the swine flu program and based upon the act or omission of a program participant in the same manner and to the same extent as the United States would be liable in any other action brought against it under such section 1346(b) and chapter 171, except that—

"(i) the liability of the United States arising out of the act or omission of a program participant may be based on any theory of liability that would govern an action against such program participant under the law of the place where the act or omission occurred, including negligence, strict liability in tort, and breach of warranty;

"(ii) the exceptions specified in section 2680(a) of title 28, United States Code, shall not apply in an action based upon the act or omission of a program participant; and

"(iii) notwithstanding section 2401(b) of title 28, United States Code, if a civil action or proceeding for personal injury or death arising out of the administration of swine flu vaccine under the swine flu program is brought within two years of the date of the administration of such vaccine and is dismissed because the plaintiff in such action or proceeding did not file an administrative claim with respect to such injury or death as required by such chapter 171, the plaintiff in such action or proceeding shall have 30 days from the date of such dismissal or two years from the date the claim arose, whichever is later, in which to file such administrative claim.   Administrative claim, filing deadline.

"(B) For purposes of this subsection, the term 'program participant' as to any particular claim means the manufacturer or distributor of the swine flu vaccine used in an inoculation under the swine flu program, the public or private agency or organization that provided an inoculation under the swine flu program without charge for such vaccine or its administration and in compliance with the   "Program participant."

Pub. Law 94-380   - 4 -   August 12, 1976

informed consent form and procedures requirements prescribed pursuant to subparagraph (F) of paragraph (1) of this subsection, and the medical and other health personnel who provided or assisted in providing an inoculation under the swine flu program without charge for such vaccine or its administration and in compliance with such informed consent form and procedures requirements.

"(3) The remedy against the United States prescribed by paragraph (2) of this subsection for personal injury or death arising out of the administration of the swine flu vaccine under the swine flu program shall be exclusive of any other civil action or proceeding for such personal injury or death against any employee of the Government (as defined in section 2671 of title 28, United States Code) or program participant whose act or omission gave raise to the claim.

Attorney General, civil action defense.   "(4) The Attorney General shall defend any civil action or proceeding brought in any court against any employee of the Government (as defined in such section 2671) or program participant (or any liability insurer thereof) based upon a claim alleging personal injury or death arising out of the administration of vaccine under the swine flu program. Any such person against whom such civil action or proceeding is brought shall deliver all process served upon him (or an attested true copy thereof) to whoever is designated by the Secretary to receive such papers, and such person shall promptly furnish copies of the pleadings and process therein to the United States attorney for the district embracing the place wherein the civil action or proceeding is brought, to the Attorney General, and to the Secretary.

"(5) (A) Upon certification by the Attorney General that a civil action or proceeding brought in any court against any employee of the Government (as defined in such section 2671) or program participant is based upon a claim alleging personal injury or death arising out of the administration of vaccine under the swine flu program, such action or proceeding shall be deemed an action against the United States under the provisions of title 28, United States Code, and all references thereto. If such action or proceeding is brought in a district court of the United States, then upon such certification the United States shall be substituted as the party defendant.

"(B) Upon a certification by the Attorney General under subparagraph (A) of this paragraph with respect to a civil action or proceeding commenced in a State court, such action or proceeding shall be removed, without bond at any time before trial, by the Attorney General to the district court of the United States of the district and division embracing the place wherein it is pending and be deemed an action brought against the United States under the provisions of title 28, United States Code, and all references thereto; and the United States shall be substituted as the party defendant. The certification of the Attorney General with respect to program participant status shall conclusively establish such status for purposes of such initial removal. Should a district court of the United States determine on a hearing on a motion to remand held before a trial on the merits that an action or proceeding is not one to which this subsection applies, the case shall be remanded to the State court.

"(C) Where an action or proceeding under this subsection is precluded because of the availability of a remedy through proceedings for compensation or other benefits from the United States as provided

August 12, 1976   - 5 -   Pub. Law 94-380

by any other law, the action or proceeding shall be dismissed, but in that event the running of any limitation of time for commencing, or filing an application or claim in, such proceedings for compensation or other benefits shall be deemed to have been suspended during the pendency of the civil action or proceeding under this subsection.

"(6) A program participant shall cooperate with the United States in the processing or defense of a claim or suit under such section 1346(b) and chapter 171 based upon alleged acts or omissions of the program participant. Upon the motion of the United States or any other party, the status as a program participant shall be revoked by the district court of the United States upon finding that the program participant has failed to so cooperate, and the court shall substitute such former participant as the party defendant in place of the United States and, upon motion, remand any such suit to the court in which it was instituted.   *Cooperation.*   *28 USC 1346, 2671 et seq.*

"(7) Should payment be made by the United States to any claimant bringing a claim under this subsection, either by way of administrative settlement or court judgment, the United States shall have, notwithstanding any provision of State law, the right to recover for that portion of the damages so awarded or paid, as well as any costs of litigation, resulting from the failure of any program participant to carry out any obligation or responsibility assumed by it under a contract with the United States in connection with the program or from any negligent conduct on the part of any program participant in carrying out any obligation or responsibility in connection with the swine flu program. The United States may maintain such action against such program participant in the district court of the United States in which such program participant resides or has its principal place of business.   *Payment.*

"(8) Within one year of the date of the enactment of the National Swine Flu Immunization Program of 1976, and semiannually thereafter, the Secretary shall submit to the Congress a report on the conduct of settlement and litigation activities under this subsection, specifying the number, value, nature, and status of all claims made thereunder, including the status of claims for recovery made under paragraph (7) of this subsection and a detailed statement of the reasons for not seeking such recovery.   *Report to Congress.*

"(l) For the purposes of subsections (j) and (k) of this section—   *Definitions.*

"(1) the phrase 'arising out of the administration' with reference to a claim for personal injury or death under the swine flu program includes a claim with respect to the manufacture or distribution of such vaccine in connection with the provision of an inoculation using such vaccine under the swine flu program;

"(2) the term 'State' includes the District of Columbia, Puerto Rico, the Virgin Islands, Guam, American Samoa, and the Trust Territory of the Pacific Islands; and

"(3) the term 'swine flu vaccine' means the vaccine against the strain of influenza virus known as influenza A/New Jersey/76 (Hsw 1N1), or a combination of such vaccine and the vaccine against the strain of influenza virus known as influenza A/Victoria/75.".

Pub. Law 94-380   - 6 -   August 12, 1976

Study.
42 USC 247b
note.

SEC. 3. The Secretary of Health, Education, and Welfare shall conduct, or provide for the conduct of, a study of the scope and extent
of liability for personal injuries or death arising out of immunization
programs and of alternative approaches to providing protection
against such liability (including a compensation system) for such

Report to
Congress.

injuries. Within one year of the date of the enactment of this Act,
the Secretary shall report to the Congress the findings of such study
and such recommendations for legislation (including proposed drafts
to carry out such recommendations) as the Secretary deems
appropriate.

Approved August 12, 1976.

LEGISLATIVE HISTORY:

SENATE REPORT No. 94-1147 (Comm. on Appropriations).
CONGRESSIONAL RECORD, Vol. 122 (1976):
    Aug. 10, considered and passed Senate and House.
WEEKLY COMPILATION OF PRESIDENTIAL DOCUMENTS, Vol. 12, No. 33:
    Aug. 12, Presidential statement.

APPENDIX D / Swine Flu Vaccine Information Forms

Important Information from the U.S. Public Health Service about Swine Flu and Victoria Flu Vaccines

INTRODUCTION

You probably have heard a good deal about swine flu and swine flu vaccine. You may know, for example, that swine flu caused an outbreak of several hundred cases at Ft. Dix, New Jersey, early in 1976- and that before then swine flu had not caused outbreaks among people since the 1920's.

With the vast majority of Americans being susceptible to swine flu, it is possible that there could be an epidemic this winter. No one can say for sure. However, if an epidemic were to break out, millions of people could get sick. Therefore, a special swine flu vaccine has been prepared and tested which should protect most people who receive it.

Certain people, such as those with chronic medical problems and the elderly, need annual protection against flu. Therefore, besides protection against swine flu, they also need protection against another type of flu (Victoria flu) that was around last winter and could occur again this winter. A separate vaccine has been prepared to give them protection against both types of flu.

These vaccines have been field tested and shown to produce very few side effects. Some people who receive the vaccine had fever and soreness during the first day or two after vaccination. These tests and past experience with other flu vaccines indicate that anything more severe than this would be highly unlikely.

Many people ask questions about flu vaccination during pregnancy. An advisory committee of the Public Health Service examined this question and reported that "there are no data specifically to contraindicate vaccination with the available killed virus vaccine in pregnancy. Women who are pregnant should be considered as having essentially the same balance of benefits and risks regarding influenza vaccination and influenza as the general population."

As indicated, some individuals will develop fever and soreness after vaccination. If you have more severe symptoms or if you have fever which lasts longer than a couple of days after vaccination, please consult your doctor or a health worker wherever you receive medical care.

While there is no reason to expect more serious reactions to this flu vaccination, persons who believe that they have been injured by this vaccination may have a claim. The Congress recently passed a law providing that such claims, with certain exceptions, may be filed only against the United States Government. Information regarding the filing of claims may be obtained by writing to the U.S. Public Health Service Claims Office, Parklawn Building, 5600 Fishers Lane, Rockville, Maryland 20852.

Attached is more information about flu and flu vaccine. Please take the time to read it carefully. You will be asked to sign a form indicating that you understand this information and that you consent to vaccination.

CDC 7.32A U.S. Department of Health, Education, and Welfare / Public Health Service / Center for Disease Control / Atlanta, Georgia 30333
8-76

160

IMPORTANT INFORMATION
ABOUT SWINE INFLUENZA (FLU) VACCINE
(MONOVALENT)

July 15, 1976

The Disease

Influenza (flu) is caused by viruses. When people get flu they may have fever, chills, headache, dry cough or muscle aches. Illness may last several days or a week or more, and complete recovery is usual. However, complications may lead to pneumonia or death in some people. For the elderly and people with diabetes or heart, lung, or kidney diseases, flu may be especially serious.

It is unlikely that you have adequate natural protection against swine flu, since it has not caused widespread human outbreaks in 45 years.

The Vaccine

The vaccine will not give you flu because it is made from killed viruses. Today's flu vaccines cause fewer side effects than those used in the past. In contrast with some other vaccines, flu vaccine can be taken safely during pregnancy.

One shot will protect most people from swine flu during the next flu season; however, either a second shot or a different dosage may be required for persons under age 25. If you are under 25 and a notice regarding such information is not attached, this information will be provided to you wherever you receive the vaccine.

Possible Vaccine Side Effects

Most people will have no side effects from the vaccine. However, tenderness at the site of the shot may occur and last for several days. Some people will also have fever, chills, headache, or muscle aches within the first 48 hours.

Special Precautions

As with any vaccine or drug, the possibility of severe or potentially fatal reactions exists. However, flu vaccine has rarely been associated with severe or fatal reactions. In some instances people receiving vaccine have had allergic reactions. You should note very carefully the following precautions:

- Children under a certain age should not routinely receive flu vaccine. Please ask about age limitations if this information is not attached.
- People with known allergy to eggs should receive the vaccine only under special medical supervision.
- People with fever should delay getting vaccinated until the fever is gone.
- People who have received another type of vaccine in the past 14 days should consult a physician before taking the flu vaccine.

If you have any questions about flu or flu vaccine, please ask.

REGISTRATION FORM

I have read the above statement about swine flu, the vaccine, and the special precautions I have had an opportunity to ask questions, including questions regarding vaccination recommendations for persons under age 25, and understand the benefits and risks of flu vaccination. I request that it be given to me or to the person named below of whom I am the parent or guardian.

INFORMATION ON PERSON TO RECEIVE VACCINE			FOR CLINIC USE
Name (Please Print)	Birthdate	Age	
Address	County of Residence		Clinic Ident.
			Date Vaccinated
			Manufacturer and Lot No.

Signature of person to receive vaccine or Parent or Guardian   Date

CDC 7.31
7-76   U.S. Department of Health, Education, and Welfare / Public Health Service / Center for Disease Control / Atlanta, Georgia 30333

IMPORTANT INFORMATION ABOUT
SWINE AND VICTORIA INFLUENZA (FLU) VACCINE
(BIVALENT)

July 15, 1976

The Disease
Influenza (flu) is caused by viruses. When people get flu they may have fever, chills, headache, dry cough or muscle aches. Illness may last several days or a week or more, and complete recovery is usual. However, complications may lead to pneumonia or death in some people. For the elderly and people with diabetes or heart, lung, or kidney diseases, flu may be especially serious.

It is unlikely that you have adequate protection against swine flu, since it has not caused widespread human outbreaks in the past 45 years. You may or may not have adequate protection against Victoria flu, although many Americans had this flu last winter. It was responsible for over 12,000 deaths.

The Vaccine
The vaccine will not give you flu because it is made from killed viruses. Today's flu vaccines cause fewer side effects than those used in the past. In contrast with some other vaccines, flu vaccine can be taken safely during pregnancy.

One shot will protect most people from swine and Victoria flu during the next flu season; however, either a second shot or a different dosage may be required for persons under age 25. If you are under 25 and a notice regarding such information is not attached, this information will be provided to you wherever you receive the vaccine.

Possible Vaccine Side Effects
Most people will have no side effects from the vaccine. However, tenderness at the site of the shot may occur and last for several days. Some people will also have fever, chills, headache, or muscle aches within the first 48 hours.

Special Precautions
As with any vaccine or drug, the possibility of severe or potentially fatal reactions exists. However, flu vaccine has rarely been associated with severe or fatal reactions. In some instances people receiving vaccine have had allergic reactions. You should note very carefully the following precautions:

- Children under a certain age should not routinely receive flu vaccine. Please ask about age limitations if this information is not attached.
- People with known allergy to eggs should receive the vaccine only under special medical supervision.
- People with fever should delay getting vaccinated until the fever is gone.
- People who have received another type of vaccine in the past 14 days should consult a physician before taking the flu vaccine.

If you have any questions about flu or flu vaccine, please ask.   ●USGPO: 1976 — 216-225

- -

REGISTRATION FORM
I have read the above statement about swine and Victoria flu, the vaccine, and the special precautions. I have had an opportunity to ask questions, including questions regarding vaccination recommendations for persons under age 25, and understand the benefits and risks of flu vaccination. I request that it be given to me or to the person named below of whom I am the parent or guardian.

INFORMATION ON PERSON TO RECEIVE VACCINE		FOR CLINIC USE
Name (Please Print)	Birthdate Age	
Address	County of Residence	Clinic Ident.
		Date Vaccinated
Signature of person to receive vaccine or Parent or Guardian Date		Manufacturer and Lot No.

CDC 7.32
7-76   U.S. Department of Health, Education, and Welfare / Public Health Service / Center for Disease Control / Atlanta, Georgia 30333

APPENDIX E

SWINE FLU OVER THE CUCKOO'S NEST

HISTORY was made last week at the annual Academy Awards night, when for the first time a single disease captured virtually every major prize given by the prestigious American Academy of Medicine. The Swine Flu virus, a relatively unknown pathogen whose last starring role was in 1918, carried off coveted "Jonases" for Best Disease, Best Symptoms, Best Virus, Best Potential Epidemic, and four other categories.

The man behind this unprecedented clinical coup is Rhinehart Glanzerman, one of the most successful of that hard-driving new breed, the pathogen press agent. At an informal press conference held after the awards ceremonies in Washington, Glanzerman gave reporters an inside look at the frenetic world of germ promotion. "It's beautiful," he told the group. "With two hundred million vaccinations booked for next season, we're out-inoculating Polio, Measles, and Smallpox combined."

Holding up a well-known flu-biz trade paper, Glanzerman pointed to a front-page story reporting overwhelming support within the medical profession for an all-out national Swine Flu vaccination program. "QUAX BACK MAX VAX!" trumpeted the headline.

"Right now we're grossing a hundred and thirty-five million at the docs' offices," the epidemic entrepreneur said with a smile, "and that's just for openers. Nothing's final yet, but our people are negotiating with the World Health Organization people for a global tour."

What do the Academy Awards really mean, Glanzerman was asked. "It's hard to say," he responded frankly. "The publicity is dynamite, and naturally it's always flattering to be honored by the people in the business. But personally I think the whole system is far too competitive. There is no *best* disease. Every parasite, every bacterium, every virus, every rickettsia has something unique to contribute. And so much of it is politics anyway. Look at Asian Flu, a real star-caliber virus if there ever was one, but it was going around during the Vietnam war. Never even *nominated.*"

What makes a star-caliber disease? "Mostly it's the name. You got a good, dirty, diseased-sounding name and you're already halfway home. Look at Gonorrhea, look at Shingles. On the other hand, take that A/Victoria Flu strain from last season. Good symptoms, good exposure, but it never made it big because it sounds like something you'd invite to tea. The public couldn't *relate.*"

Another reporter wanted to know if the fact that Swine Flu started out in another medium — namely, hogs — detracted in any way from its claim to greatness.

"Not in the least," the energetic agent shot back. "Hoof-and-Mouth, Elephantiasis, Rabies — all of them began in other media. You judge a human disease by how it stands up in humans. If some pig wants to claim credit, let him try and sue."

Why has Swine Flu been such a hit?

"Like I said, I think it's because Swine Flu is a disease that people can relate to. Headache, nausea, fever — nothing too deep, symptom wise. It's not trying to be the new Yellow Fever. I mean, the average Joe looks at some of these exotic diseases you see being promoted and he's lost. Sure it's awful, he says but what does it have to do with me? With Swine Flu you don't have to have an M.D. to understand what's going on. It reaches a mass audience and brings a little misery into their lives."

How did Swine Flu make it big?

"I played the nostalgia angle," Glanzerman said. "These last few seasons have been all revivals anyway, and I figured the Swine was a natural.

"But nothing happens overnight in this business. Last year I made the rounds of all the big agencies — N.I.H., H.E.W., even the A.M.A. — and not one of them would touch it. Everywhere it was the same story: Come back when you've had some national exposure. Well, Rhinehart Glanzerman doesn't discourage so easy. I figured if we opened out in the sticks and got a little local excitement going it would be contagious. And it paid off. Our début was a smash, we got a few rave notices, and the rest," beamed the influenza impresario, "is epideminology."

— RICHARD LEIBMANN-SMITH

**THE NEW YORKER
MAY 31, 1976**

Notes

1. R. E. Neustadt, and H. V. Fineberg, *The Swine Flu Affair: Decision-Making on a Slippery Disease* (Washington, D.C.: U.S. Department of Health, Education and Welfare, 1978).
2. In one of those strange coincidences of history, on the very day that the swine flu virus was identified at the CDC, the *New York Times* carried an Op Ed article on influenza by Dr. Edwin Kilbourne, one of the world's leading influenza experts. The chief proponent of the theory that influenza returns in periodic eleven-year cycles, he pointed out that the time was rapidly approaching when a new influenza pandemic might be expected. He "urgently suggest[ed] that those concerned with public health had best plan without further delay for an imminent natural disaster" *(New York Times,* February 13, 1976, p. 33). Both Kilbourne's ideas and Kilbourne himself would play a major role in subsequent developments in the swine flu affair.
3. Erwin H. Ackerknecht, *History and Geography of the Most Important Diseases* (New York: Hafner, 1965). For more general information, see F. H. Garrison, *An Introduction to the History of Medicine* (Philadelphia: Saunders, 1917), and A. Castiglioni, *A History of Medicine* (New York: Knopf, 1947).
4. William H. McNeill, *Plagues and Peoples* (New York: Doubleday, 1976). The general reader should be aware that McNeill's book has come under serious attack by professional historians of medicine, who accuse him of playing fast and loose with historical facts. McNeill, on the other hand, accuses the professionals of pedantic narrowness of view and of neglecting the "big picture" that he champions. In any event, the book makes very good reading and stimulates thought in many areas.
5. John Farley, *The Spontaneous Generation Controversy: From Descartes to Oparin* (Baltimore: Johns Hopkins University Press, 1974).
6. Charles Rosenberg, *The Cholera Years* (Chicago: University of Chicago Press, 1962). See also Erwin H. Ackerknecht, "Anticontagionism between 1821 and 1867," *Bulletin of the History of Medicine* 22 (1948):562–93.
7. G. Miller, *The Adoption of Inoculation for Smallpox in England and France* (Philadelphia: University of Pennsylvania Press, 1959).
8. Smallpox is almost the only infectious disease of humans to which the term *eradication* can reasonably be applied. This is because it is unique in being confined exclusively to man, with no animal reservoirs like influenza in birds and horses or anthrax in cattle. Further, it spreads only from human to human, with no intermediate living vectors, such as the mosquito for malaria and yellow fever, the rat louse for plague, or the snail for schistosomiasis. Individual immunity in smallpox is also thoroughly effective and long-lasting. The strategy employed in the WHO smallpox eradication campaign was therefore not to attempt vaccination of the entire world's population, which would be technically difficult, but rather

165

to identify every individual case of smallpox, and then to isolate it by building around it a wall of vaccinated individuals, to inhibit further spread. With the cooperation of health officials throughout the world, this strategy proved highly effective, and the last natural case of smallpox was reported in 1977.

9. W.I.B. Beveridge, *Influenza: The Last Great Plague* (New York: Prodist, 1977). For other histories of early influenza, see T. Thompson, *Annals of Influenza* (London: Sydenham Society, 1852), and C. Creighton, *A History of Epidemics in Britain* (London: Cambridge University Press, 1894).

10. "Glimpses of Influenza in the Past," *British Medical Journal* 1 (1919):138. Concerning "the newe acquayntance," see T. Francis, Jr., "Influenza: The New Acquayntance," *Annals of Internal Medicine* 39 (1953):203.

11. Noah Webster, cited in Adolph A. Hoehling, *The Great Epidemic* (Boston: Little Brown, 1961), p. 6

12. W.I.B. Beveridge, *Influenza: The Last Great Plague.*

13. Edwin D. Kilbourne, "Epidemiology of Influenza," in *The Influenza Viruses and Influenza* ed., Edwin D. Kilbourne, (New York: Academic Press, 1975), pp. 483–538.

14. C. A. Gill, *The Genesis of Epidemics* (London: Balliere, Tindall, and Cox, 1928). C. H. Andrewes has suggested (in *Perspectives in Virology*, ed., M. Pollard [New York: Wiley, 1959], pp. 184–96) that Central Asia may serve as a reservoir of animal influenza strains of importance for human disease.

15. Perhaps the best general description of the 1918–19 pandemic is that written by Alfred W. Crosby, Jr. *(Epidemic and Peace, 1918* [Westport, Conn.: Greenwood Press, 1976]). Of somewhat more limited value, but interesting for their anecdotal remembrances, are Richard Collier's *The Plague of the Spanish Lady* (New York: Atheneum, 1974), and Hoehling's, *The Great Epidemic.*

16. Edwin D. Kilbourne, *The Influenza Viruses and Influenza,* pp. 483–538.

17. *Summary Report of Conference on Influenza Vaccine Activity for 1977–78.* U.S. Public Health Service, Department of Health, Education, and Welfare, March 21, 1977. Other information on the economic costs of influenza may be found in the Proceedings of Influenza Workshop, no. 4, U.S. Public Health Service, Department of Health, Education, and Welfare, 1973.

18. Much of the following discussion of the 1957–58 pandemic was recorded in an unpublished monograph on the subject by Horace G. Ogden, who was involved in the program firsthand at the Center for Disease Control. I wish to thank the CDC and Mr. Ogden for permission to use this material.

19. This account of the February 14, 1976, meeting was put together from personal interviews with Sencer, Meyer, Seal, and many persons on the CDC staff, held during the fall of 1979. The reader may wonder at the precision with which the participants appeared to recall the events at this and many other meetings, some three and one-half years afterward. It should be recalled, however, that not only had they all been interviewed for the Neustadt and Fineberg report *The Swine Flu Affair,* but they all had spent many hours recently reviewing their documents and their memories, in connection with the giving of depositions in the lawsuits that followed termination of the program.

20. "Influenza Workshop," transcript of meeting at Bethesda, Maryland, on February 20, 1976, sponsored jointly by the Center for Disease Control, the Bureau of Biologics, and the National Institute of Allergy and Infectious Diseases, U.S. Public Health Service, Department of Health, Education, and Welfare.

21. S. Shoenbaum; B. McNeil; and J. Kavet, "The Swine Influenza Decision," *New England Journal of Medicine* 295 (1976):759–65.

22. Much later, Hattwicke would raise the ire of the entire scientific community by claim-

ing that he had specifically warned the ACIP meeting that Guillain-Barré disease might accompany swine flu immunization. No other participant at the meeting can recall such a warning, nor does the prior medical literature appear to hint at a relationship. Hattwicke persists in his contention, and in October 1979, when questioned by interviewer Mike Wallace on the television show *Sixty Minutes,* came close to calling Sencer a liar for claiming that the warning had not been issued.

23. All three of the persons involved remembered the mention of this subject, and in substantially similar terms, at the separate personal interviews conducted for the preparation of this report.

24. Summary Minutes of Meeting, Immunization Practices Advisory Committee, March 10, 1976, Center for Disease Control, Atlanta, Georgia, p. 5.

25. This is a personal assessment of these individuals, gained during extensive interviews, but substantially confirmed by other participants. David Mathew's recollections of the affair, recorded in these pages, were similarly obtained during a personal interview.

26. Quoted by Neustadt and Fineberg, *The Swine Flu Affair.*

27. *Weekly Compilation of Presidential Documents* 12, no. 3, (March 29, 1976), pp. 483-84.

28. An excellent review of immunity in influenza infection can be found in J. L. Schulman, "Immunology of Influenza," in *The Influenza Viruses and Influenza,* ed. E. D. Kilbourne, pp. 373-93.

29. T. Francis, Jr., "Influenza: The New Acquayntance."

30. R. G. Webster, and W. G. Laver, "Antigenic Variation of Influenza Viruses," in Kilbourne, ed., *The Influenza Viruses and Influenza,* pp. 269-314.

31. B. C. Easterday, "Animal Influenza," in Kilbourne, ed., *The Influenza Viruses and Influenza,* pp. 449-81.

32. See n. 8.

33. U.S., Congress, House, Subcommittee on Health and the Environment of the Committee on Interstate and Foreign Commerce, *Hearings on Proposed National Swine Flu Immunization Program,* 94th Cong., 2d sess., 1976.

34. Ibid.

35. U.S., Congress, Senate, Subcommittee on Health of the Committee on Labor and Public Welfare, *Hearings on Swine Flu Immunization Program,* 94th Cong., 2d sess., 1976.

36. U.S., Congress, House, Committee on Appropriations, *Emergency Supplemental Appropriations, 1976,* House Report 94-1004, 94th Cong., 2d sess., 1976.

37. U.S., Congress, House, *Congressional Record,* 94th Cong., 2d sess., 1976, pp. 2861-65; 2871-75.

38. U.S., Congress, Senate, *Congressional Record,* 94th Cong., 2d sess., 1976, 5347-56.

39. U.S., Congress, Senate, Committee on Appropriations, *Emergency Supplemental Appropriations, 1976,* Senate Report 94-0000, 94th Cong., 2d sess., 1976.

40. U.S. Senate, *Congressional Record,* 94th Cong., 2d sess., 1976, pp. 5347-56.

41. *Weekly Compilation of Presidential Documents* 12, no. 16, (April 19, 1976), p. 656.

42. The foregoing account of the personality and bureaucratic interactions among the participants was distilled from comments made during personal interviews with Mathews, Cooper, Sencer, Meyer, and Seal in HEW, and with Harold Schmeck of the *New York Times.*

43. Philip M. Boffey, "Swine Flu Campaign: Should We Vaccinate the Pigs?" *Science* 192 (1976):870.

44. World Health Organization, "Influenza," *Weekly Epidemiological Record* 51 (April 15, 1976):123.

45. *Lancet,* July 3, 1976, pp. 4–5; 25–26; and 31–32.

46. Transcript of Workshop on Swine Flu Field Trials. National Institute of Allergy and Infectious Diseases, Bethesda, Maryland, June 21, 1976. The results are summarized by P. D. Parkman; G. J. Galasso; F. H. Top; and G. R. Noble, *Journal of Infectious Diseases* 134 (1976):100.

47. Philip M. Boffey, "Swine Flu Vaccine: A Component is Missing." *Science* 193 (1976): 1224.

48. *New York Times,* editorials, February 23, April 6, June 8, and August 9, 1976.

49. Edwin M. Kilbourne, *New York Times,* April 14, August 9, 1976.

50. J. Enders; T. C. Chalmers; R. H. Ebert; J. T. Grayston; A. Lilienfeld; and D. D. Rutstein, *New York Times,* January 10, 1977.

51. Morris would later be fired from his job at BoB, a move that led to years of argument and litigation. Morris would claim that the action was unjust and a punishment for his dissent, whereas BoB would claim that the discharge was for just cause, and that Morris was a poor scientist. The controversy is detailed by Philip M. Boffey, in *Science* 194 (1976):1021.

52. "Stockpiling of Monovalent Influenza A/New Jersey/76 Influenza Vaccine," Center for Disease Control Memorandum, Atlanta, Georgia June 7, 1976.

53. *Davis* v. *Wyeth Laboratories, Inc.,* 339 F. 2nd 121 (9th Cir. 1968), and *Reyes* v. *Wyeth Laboratories, Inc.,* 498 F. 2nd 1264 (5th Cir. 1974).

54. U.S., Congress, House, Subcommittee on Health and the Environment of the Committee on Interstate and Foreign Commerce, *Supplemental Hearings on Swine Flu Immunization Program,* 94th Cong., 2d sess., 1976.

55. It is unfortunate that this remarkable meeting took place "off the record," so that no transcript exists, as is the case in formal subcommittee sessions. The author did attend, in order to monitor the proceedings on behalf of the Senate Health Subcommittee.

56. *Weekly Compilation of Presidential Documents,* 12, no. 30, (July 19, 1976), p. 1180.

57. *Supplemental Hearings on Swine Flu Immunization Program,* 94th Cong., 2d sess., 1976.

58. U.S., Congress, House, Subcommittee on Consumer Protection and Finance of the Committee on Interstate and Foreign Commerce, *Hearing on Legionnaires' Disease,* 94th Cong., 2d sess., 1976.

59. A useful summary of the initial failure to identify Legionnaires' Disease, and of the final solution to the problem, was made by B. J. Culliton, "Legion Fever: Postmortem on an Investigation That Failed," *Science* 194 (1976):1025, and idem, "Legion Fever: 'Failed' Investigation May Be Successful after All," *Science* 195 (1977):469.

60. *Weekly Compilation of Presidential Documents,* 12, no. 32, August 6, 1976, p. 1249.

61. U.S., Congress, Senate, Committee on Appropriations, *National Swine Flu Immunization Program of 1976,* Senate Report 94–1147, 94th Cong., 2d sess., 1976.

62. U.S., Congress, Senate, *Congressional Record,* 94th Cong., 2d sess., 1976, pp. 14108–118.

63. U.S., Congress, House, *Congressional Record,* 94th Cong., 2d sess., 1976, pp. 8644–45.

64. Ibid, pp. 8649–54.

65. "The Swine Flu Program: An Unprecedented Venture in Preventive Medicine." Report to the Congress by the Comptroller General of the United States (General Accounting Office), June 27, 1977. This report is also appended to the

House of Representatives oversight hearing on swine flu of September 16, 1977 (U.S., Congress, House, Subcommittee on Interstate and Foreign Commerce, *Hearing on Review and Evaluation of the Swine Flu Immunization Program,* 95 Cong., 1st sess., 1977.). It provides an excellent summary of the many problems faced by the Immunization Program from its very inception.

66. The Pittsburgh incident demonstrated once again that no matter how improbable an event may be, it remains *possible* and cannot be ruled out. The ensuing debate also demonstrated that "experts" will always be found who are willing to argue forcefully on one side or the other of any issue of public concern. This is brought out well, in this case, by Philip M. Boffey, "Swine Flu: Were the Three Deaths in Pittsburgh a Coincidence?" *Science* 194 (1976):590.

67. B. Cunningham, *New York Post,* October 14, 1976, p. 2. The *Post* ran a story some weeks later (October 25) suggesting that mobster Carlo Gambino had been the object of a Mafia "hit," for which the mode of execution was reputed to have been the swine flu shot he is thought to have received not long before his death!

68. D. M. Rubin, V. Hendy, "Swine Influenza and the News Media," *Annals of Internal Medicine,* 87 (1977):769.

69. "Administration of the National Swine Flu Immunization Program of 1976. Final Report to Congress." U.S. Department of Health, Education and Welfare, 1978. In this report is a breakdown of vaccine coverage of the population, and of the full costs of the program.

70. Ibid.

71. Ibid.

72. U.S., Congress, Senate, Subcommittee on Health of the Committee on Labor and Public Welfare, *Hearing on Suspension of the Swine Flu Immunization Program, 1976,* 94th Cong., 2d sess., 1976, p. 10.

73. F. Leneman, "The Guillain-Barré Syndrome." *Archives of Internal Medicine* 118 (1966):139.

74. *Hearing on Suspension of the Swine Flu Immunization Program, 1976,* 94th Cong., 2d sess., 1976, p. 10.

75. Department of Health, Education and Welfare Press Release, December 16, 1976.

76. *Summary Report of Conference on Influenza Vaccine Activity for 1977-78,* U.S. Public Health Service, Department of Health, Education, and Welfare, March 21, 1977.

77. Ibid.

78. Ibid.

79. *Hearing on Suspension of the Swine Flu Immunization Program, 1976,* 94th Cong., 2d sess., 1976, p. 10.

80. Ibid.

81. Harry Schwartz, "The Swine Flu Fiasco," *New York Times,* December 21, 1976.

82. See, for example, T. O'Toole, "Why The Swine Flu Program Failed," *Washington Post,* January 30, 1977, p. C-3; and G. A. Silver, "Lessons of the Swine Flu Debacle," *The Nation* (February 12, 1977): p. 166. Others, and especially virologist Kilbourne, attempted to defend the program; see Edwin D. Kilbourne, "Influenza Pandemic in Perspective," *Journal American Medical Association* 237 (1977):1225; idem, "Swine Flu: The Virus That Vanished," *Human Nature* (March 1979):68; and the Enders et al. letter to the *Times* referred to in Chapt. 8, n. 9.

83. "Summary Report on Influenza Virus Vaccine Use," U.S. Public Health Service, Department of Health, Education and Welfare, February 7, 1977.

84. *Summary Report of Conference on Influenza Vaccine Activity for 1977–78.*

85. U.S., Congress, House, Subcommittee on Health and the Environment of the Committee on Interstate and Foreign Commerce, *Hearing on Review and Evaluation of the Swine Flu Immunization Program,* 95th Cong., 1st sess., 1977.

86. "Administration of the National Swine Flu Immunization Program of 1976." Final Report to Congress, U.S. Department of Health, Education, and Welfare, 1978.

87. Department of Health, Education and Welfare, *Reports and Recommendations of the National Immunization Work Groups,* March 11, 1977.

88. HEW report to Congress on vaccine liability issues, November 1977.

89. "Administration of the National Swine Flu Immunization Program of 1976."

90. R. E. Neustadt and H. V. Fineberg, *The Swine Flu Affair: Decision-Making on a Slippery Disease.*

Selected Readings

The Science of Influenza

Beveridge, W.I.B. *Influenza: The Last Great Plague*. London: Heinemann, 1977. A very brief but excellent nontechnical discussion of the biology of the influenza virus and the epidemiology of the disease.

Kilbourne, Edwin D., ed. *The Influenza Viruses and Influenza*. New York: Academic Press, 1975.

Stuart-Harris, Charles H., and Schild, Geoffrey C. *Influenza: The Viruses and the Disease*. Littleton, Mass.: Publishing Sciences Group, 1976.

Selby, Philip, ed. *Influenza: Virus, Vaccine, and Strategy*. New York: Academic Press, 1976.

All three of these volumes are highly technical, but provide a thorough review of contemporary knowledge of the virus, the disease, and immunization strategies.

The History of Influenza

Creighton, Charles. *A History of Epidemics in Britain*. London: Cambridge University Press, 1894. A classic text, still of great use and interest to the student of influenza.

Beveridge, W.I.B. *Influenza: The Last Great Plague*. London: Heineman, 1977. In addition to a useful summary of the science, Beveridge provides the general reader with the best brief summary of its history.

Crosby, Alfred W., Jr. *Epidemic and Peace, 1918*. Westport Conn.: Greenwood Press, 1976. This is the best comprehensive account of the influenza pandemic of 1918–19, told in a highly readable style.

Swine Flu, 1976

Neustadt, Richard E., and Fineberg, Harvey V. *The Swine Flu Affair: Decision-Making on a Slippery Disease*. Washington, D.C.: U.S. Department of Health, Education, and Welfare, 1978. This is a comprehensive study, which examines the entire venture in all its detail. It provides an invaluable reference source for the events of 1976.

Osborne, June, ed. *Influenza in America 1918–1976.* New York: Prodist, 1977. The proceedings of a symposium held by the American Association for the History of Medicine. Excepting only an excellent and comprehensive chapter by Arthur J. Viseltear on the congressional politics of swine flu, the volume is not very useful.

Boffey, Philip M., wrote a series of four articles in *Science*: May 14, 1976, pp. 636–41; August 13, 1976, pp. 559–63; September 24, 1976, pp. 1224–25; January 14, 1977, pp. 155–59. Also, "Soft Evidence and Hard Sell," *New York Times Magazine,* September 5, 1976, p. 8. This is a superb series of contemporary discussions and commentary on the developing swine flu affair, written for both scientists and laymen.

U.S. Congress. Senate. Subcommittee on Health of Committee on Labor and Public Welfare. *Hearing on Swine Flu Immunization Program.* 94th Cong., 2d Sess., 1976. A useful introduction to the swine flu immunization program, the administration's bases for its adoption, and its goals.

U.S. Congress. House. Subcommittee on Health and the Environment, Committee on Interstate and Foreign Commerce. *Supplemental Hearings on Swine Flu Immunization Program.* 94th Cong., 2d Sess., 1976. An excellent review of the problems of insurance liability on swine flu vaccines and attempts to solve them.

General Accounting Office. *The Swine Flu Program: An Unprecedented Venture in Preventive Medicine. Report to the Congress by the Comptroller General of the United States, 1977.* (Reprinted in U.S. Congress. House. Subcommittee on Health and the Environment, Committee on Interstate and Foreign Commerce. *Hearing on Review and Evaluation of the Swine Flu Immunization Program.* 95th Cong., 1st Sess., 1977). This study reviews the planning and operation of the National Influenza Immunization Program, with an emphasis on technical and contractual problems, and gives recommendations for future efforts of this type. The House *Hearing* of September 16, 1977, expands upon this examination.

The Politics of Health

Redman, Eric. *The Dance of Legislation.* New York: Simon and Schuster, 1973. A delightful account of the workings of the legislative process on a health issue, by a Senate staffer.

Strickland, Stephen P. *Politics, Science, and Dread Disease. A Short History of United States Medical Research Policy.* Cambridge, Mass.: Harvard University Press, 1972. The fascinating political story of how and why the U.S. government became active in health research, with many instructive insights into the workings of the American political process.

Greenberg, Daniel S. *The Politics of Pure Science. An Inquiry into the Relationship between Science and Government in the United States.* New York: New American Library, 1967. Greenberg does for the physical sciences what Strickland does for biomedical science. An informative study of the structure of "big science" and how it interacts with big government.

Index